Downs Children

The Story of Roland

Downs Children

The Story of Roland

Robert Anderson

Zambezi Publishing Ltd

First published in 2023 in the UK by Zambezi Publishing Ltd
Plymouth, Devon PL2 2EQ
Tel: +44 (0)1752 367 300
email: zambezipub@gmail.com   www.zampub.com

British Library Cataloguing in Publication Data:
A catalogue record for this book is available from the British Library

ISBN: 978-1-903065-73-0
Photographs copyright © 2023 Robert Anderson
Typesetting by Zambezi Publishing Ltd, Plymouth

About the Author

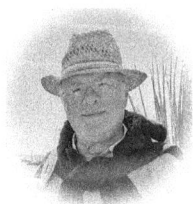

Both from North London originally, Robert and Pat met and married in the early 1970s, by which time Pat already had two sons from her first marriage. Launching into family life straightaway, Robert and Pat had two boys together in quick succession, the second of whom – Roland – was born in 1976 with Downs Syndrome.

This book tells the story of Roland's upbringing, a 44-year caring marathon that had its joys and rewards but also taxed his parents' emotional and physical resources to their limits.

Contents

Foreword

Writing this book in my early seventies, I am looking back on 44 years of caring for my son Roland who has Downs Syndrome. Sadly, severe dementia prevents my wife Pat from contributing to the book – though she was devoted to Roland's care until illness overtook her.

This is not only a 'how-to' guide for parenting a Downs child. It also explores the impact of ageing and illness on parents and carers, and the support available from local authorities and the NHS for Downs people and those who care for them. If, as a parent, you continue caring until you are elderly, your health may begin to fail whilst you are still 'in harness'. You will then come up against the discrepancies between governmental and NHS provision for congenitally disabled adults versus that for the mainstream elderly. In brief, Downs children and others who are 'statemented' as having substantial special needs are entitled to special education and potentially lifetime care at the expense of the local authority. In contrast, pensioners who were born healthy are generally expected to self-fund their care as geriatrics. The increasing incidence of dementia in the UK's ageing population, and the attempts to manage it, make this a very topical issue.

I hope that Roland's story will inform and encourage those who are parents and carers for children and adults who share his condition. In the aftermath of Roland's birth, I remember how helpful it was not only to learn that organizations like The Downs Syndrome Association and satellite groups existed but also to read the factual yet very human accounts of their life experiences written by other parents in this situation.

1: What is Downs Syndrome?

Downs Syndrome is a relatively common chromosomal abnormality that causes learning difficulties and can affect physical development. It can also cause other health issues. Around one child in 600 is born with Downs, and there are around 750 such births annually in the UK. About 60,000 people with Downs Syndrome are estimated to live in the UK.

The syndrome affects each person differently, so the learning difficulties can vary in scope and severity. For example, some children with the condition attend mainstream schools. Downs Syndrome slows a child's mental and social development and usually limits it to a significant extent. However, with the right support, they can be expected to lead an active life with a degree of independence, and some adults with Downs are in regular employment.

The condition is commonly associated with specific physical and facial features, but like everyone else, people with Downs vary in appearance and have inherited family traits. A proportion of people with Downs will also experience difficulties such as heart conditions and increased susceptibility to infections. In the past, such complications generally led to reduced life expectancy, but advances in treatment and care mean people with Downs can now expect to live into their sixties.

What Causes Downs Syndrome?

When a baby is conceived, it inherits the genetic coding for its physical structure from its parents in the form of 46 chromosomes – 23 from each parent. Downs Syndrome is associated with a fault in chromosome No. 21 which appears as an abnormal additional chromosome.

What is Downs Syndrome?

How Common is Downs Syndrome?

Any woman can have a child with Downs, although the chances increase with age. At the age of 20, the chance is about 1 in 1,400; at 30, the probability increases to 1 in 1,000, but at 40 years, the chance is 1 in 100, and by 45, the odds are 1 in 20. Paternal age can also be a contributory factor if the father is over 40 years old. Having said this, more children with Downs are born to women under 35 years of age – but this is considered to be due to their greater fertility than those who are older.

Can Downs Syndrome be Detected Before Birth?

Yes – there are screening tests and diagnostic tests. In simple terms, screening using blood tests or ultrasound examinations can indicate the probability of abnormalities such as Downs – but these tests are not definitive. Diagnostic tests such as chorionic villus sampling (CVS) from the placenta, amniocentesis (from the fluid surrounding the baby), and percutaneous umbilical blood sampling (PUBS) give a much more dependable result. Still, there is a small risk of these procedures leading to miscarriage.

Can Downs Syndrome be Cured?

At present, there is no cure. However, nowadays, there is improved societal inclusion and acceptance of people with Downs, with mainstream education having a big part to play. So, despite the availability of fairly reliable and safe screening and diagnostic tests, many women decide not to terminate their pregnancies despite a positive test for Downs Syndrome. As a result, and owing to the greater number of women waiting until their late thirties before having children, the incidence of the condition is increasing in the UK.

For more detailed information about Downs Syndrome, I recommend the Downs Syndrome Association at www.downs-syndrome.org.uk and the NHS at www.nhs.uk. The USA also has relevant sites, e.g., www.ndss.org.

2: Roland's Early Life

My wife Pat's and my families both hail from Islington, North London. My dad was a teacher. Pat's dad was a gas fitter. Our mothers were both housewives who occasionally took part-time jobs. I met Pat after her first marriage broke up. She had returned home from Cornwall with her two sons, William and Patrick, aged nine and seven years. Her younger brother James had been a school friend of mine, and I was a regular visitor to their parental home near Finsbury Park. Pat is ten years my senior, but there was an instant sense of 'recognition' and attraction when we met, so the age difference didn't seem to matter. Our relationship developed rapidly. Pat needed a home for herself and her sons, so she found secretarial work and started to save. William opted to live with his dad in Devon when her divorce came through. I pooled my finances with Pat, and we bought a small house in Kettering, Northants - eighty miles north of London – and moved there with Patrick in September 1973. We were married two months later. We wanted to have children, but Pat had toxaemia of pregnancy when carrying William at the age of 24, and Patrick was born heavily jaundiced when he arrived three years later. Moreover, since Pat was in her late thirties when we were considering an addition to the family, we couldn't ignore the potential risks to her and a new baby. It was, therefore, a relief when our first child – Warren – arrived healthy in every respect. Reassured by this, we decided to have a second child to be a companion for him – as his brother, Patrick, was ten years older.

Roland's Birth
Pat fell pregnant aged forty, and Patrick voiced his concern that the baby might be 'Mongol' – as Downs Syndrome used to be called then. Pat and I pooh-poohed the suggestion – partly

because Warren had turned out healthy and partly because we didn't want to countenance it. Shortly afterwards, I noticed a large black book in the local library titled 'Downs Syndrome' in gold lettering. I hadn't heard of this term in those days and continued browsing. (More about this book later.)

In the mid-1970s, there was no screening test for Downs. There was a diagnostic test becoming available in our local area, but Pat's pregnancy was by then too advanced for termination to be an option, and anyway, Pat was against abortion.

Doctors rang no alarm bells as the pregnancy progressed, and Roland was born in the same local hospital as Warren at full term after a short and uneventful labour. All skin and bones and jaundiced, he looked like a little old man. Apart from this, he didn't look unusual to us, and his birth weight was a regular 3.4 kg. However, I noticed looks of concern exchanged by the nurses, but nothing was said, and we were allowed to take him home. Pat remarked that Patrick had been born jaundiced and Roland probably just needed 'feeding up'.

Infancy - Age 0-4 Years

A few days later, our GP made a home visit and broke the news that Roland was generally healthy, but a blood test had revealed he had Downs Syndrome – trisomy 21. The doctor was sympathetic and did his best to be positive and informative, but Pat and I were deeply shocked by the short and long-term implications. Roland was a child who would need a lot of extra care, and he might never properly grow up.

Pat felt she had somehow let me down. She had given me a damaged baby. She felt that Roland wasn't her real baby. He was something like a changeling in a fairy story. I didn't feel this way but was apprehensive about the future. Roland's birth was a life-changing event for the whole family. Our family life together had started so positively, but now our dreams and plans had been knocked sideways. Patrick's fears had been realized. He didn't want anything to do with Roland; he seemed to regard Roland as a non-person, and this attitude didn't change until Roland was much older. At only two years of age, Warren simply accepted that he had a new brother. He didn't seem to feel side-lined or disadvantaged by the additional care and attention Roland needed from Pat and me. Warren and Roland slept in the same room, so they got to know each other from day one.

The acute feelings of devastation and helplessness quickly began to be eclipsed by the realization that Roland needed us to step up to the plate. Pat was an experienced mother, and her skills kicked in. Roland was not diagnosed with any heart or breathing problems but was low in muscle tone and 'floppy'- initially less responsive than a normal baby to sensory input. He lay and snuffled instead of crying when hungry. It would have been easy for Pat and me to sleep through his feebly expressed need for night-feeding, but Pat was alert to the slightest signs of restlessness and responded to these. Roland was also inefficient at breastfeeding, and his erratic swallowing reflex made him prone to dribbling his milk or choking. He did better with bottles of formula milk. His body-temperature regulation was poor, so we had to take extra care to prevent him from becoming chilled or over-hot. The latter was an issue because Roland was born in August 1976 – the hottest UK summer for 100 years – which was very appropriate for the Chinese Year of the Fire Dragon! That year, my brother was up at Cambridge Uni and regularly visited. At the end of his August visit, I saw him off on his return train journey at 10:30 pm – it was dark, but the temperature at Kettering station was 84F!

At that time, stories about cot-deaths were making the news. We made sure Roland and Warren had 'breathable' mattresses and pillows. Warren was a lively 21 months-old toddler when Roland was born, so we did our best to ensure he got all the love and attention he needed too.

Despite the combination of breast and bottle feeding, Roland initially failed to put on weight. We started him on milky porridge despite reading that babies with Downs could be prone to intestinal blockages if given solids too early. In Roland's case, it worked. His jaundice cleared up, and he began to put on weight. However, I would not advise parents to feed their babies any non-standard diets or supplements without the approval of a qualified medical practitioner.

Owing to Roland's special needs, we received more attention from health visitors and our GP than normal. Their input regarding feeding, diet, weight and developmental milestones was generally welcome and helpful. Even a session with a rather 'superior' consultant, surrounded by student doctors, turned out to include good advice. His suggestion that we join support groups seemed to us at the time rather a cop-out by a medical profession that still tended to write children with Downs Syndrome off as incurable and to send their parents on a guilt-trip. But on reflection we looked at the options and discovered The Downs Babies Association (later renamed The Downs Syndrome Association).

The Downs Babies Association, then headed by Rex Brinkworth, put us in touch with a local parents' group and we attended some of its meetings. Most of the mums and dads were of early middle age but there was one 25-year-old mum of a Downs child there who was thinking of having another baby. There were visiting speakers, some of whom gave useful information on claiming benefits and how to make a will in favour of a child who lacked financial capacity. Speakers also acquainted us with common issues around health and physical development. Downs was associated with certain physical 'stigmata' including short stature, slanted eyes, protruding tongue, and small clumsy hands with short fingers. However, these were by no means universal, and some children were only mildly affected. In Roland's case he did have low muscle tone, hyper-extensible joints and a tendency to let his tongue protrude. He also became chilled or too hot rather easily. Downs certainly also entailed learning difficulties and sometimes other psychological issues nowadays labelled as Autism and Asperger's but on an emotional level there was usually a fairly placid nature with a capacity to relate to others.

Rex Brinkworth was a strong advocate for treating babies with Downs Syndrome as normally as possible. He had a daughter with Downs. She had been born in France where Rex and his wife had been told by a doctor that their baby would be a legume (a vegetable) for the rest of her life. Rex's daughter was to disprove this opinion in spectacular fashion. Francoise reportedly developed many skills: she passed her driving test, learned to read music and play the piano, became fluent in French, and lived independently in a flat!

One of the keys to optimizing development was to ignore floppiness and passivity and instead press forward with a programme of gentle but persistent stimulation: tactile, auditory and visual. We soon discovered that Roland was looking at his surroundings with apparent interest and at bedtime he enjoyed lying in his cot watching and listening to a clockwork mobile that rotated above him and played nursery rhyme tunes.

I frequented the local library and read all the books I could find about the experiences of parents with Downs babies. It was on one such visit that I again caught sight of the large black book with gold lettering. Its actual title wasn't 'Downs Syndrome' – it was 'The Backward Child' by Sir Cyril Burt. Evidently my first encounter with the book had been an omen.

The accounts of parenting varied widely in their tone and content. Some related rather desperate struggles with what was felt to be the nearly impossible burden of an impaired and sometimes unresponsive child with no prospect of progress or release. Others told the poignant story of their child also having been born with a heart defect that led to death in infancy or childhood. It didn't help that there was still a presumption in some quarters that handicapped children should be 'put away' and live out their lives in institutions. Worse still, the news media carried stories of babies rejected by their parents because of Downs Syndrome being given 'nursing care only' in hospitals and effectively starved to death. Whistleblowing nurses exposed this practice, and it was stopped.

But some parents told a happier tale: their son or daughter gained a basic education, developed social skills and even held down a simple job. In all the books I read about parenting a child with Downs, it was the mother that seemed to be more affected. Pat was no exception. The joy of bringing a child into the world was tempered with worry about his future and her ability to care for him. It wasn't so challenging for me. I was deeply saddened by the situation – and helped support Pat as best I could – but needed to concentrate on improving my job prospects as we were rather short of money in the early years at Kettering.

Pat even talked about having another baby – as if to overlay the 'failure'. But, as the initial shock and grief subsided, common sense prevailed and there was no more talk of another addition to the family.

Within our extended family reactions to Roland's arrival varied. My brother and Pat's brother, James, were curious but emotionally detached. Our respective parents were initially shocked and sympathetic but as our regular visits to London resumed, they soon got used to Roland who to them seemed much the same as a normal baby in his behaviour. One of our neighbours was a nurse and he took a look at Roland. He opined that Roland didn't seem too severely affected by Downs Syndrome compared with others in his experience.

There was plenty of literature about special education, with developmental checklists and milestones for use by both teachers and parents. There was a particularly long list of these aimed at the 0-4 years age group including self-help skills, social skills, physical development, cognitive development and language development. Children who were not learning-disabled would be expected to pass all these milestones, but Downs children might struggle with them.

To stimulate visually: bright objects, mobiles, pictures, toys and moving objects were recommended – as was propping the child up to see familiar people and surroundings. Auditory stimulation could be from toys and objects which made different sounds, plus talking and singing to the child. Tactile experience could be broadened using toys that were soft, furry or fluffy, smooth or rough.

In terms of physical development, we encouraged Roland to push with arms and legs, turn his head, roll over, reach for and grasp objects. Following on from this it was useful for him to practise holding then releasing, placing objects inside and upon others, putting pieces together and taking them apart, building with bricks, stacking cups. A baby bouncer was used to strengthen his legs and accustom Roland to an upright position – though of course it was expected that he would go through a crawling stage before developing sufficient balance to stand unaided.

Communication was important too. Cues to look out for included smiling, cooing, following objects or sounds with the eyes, reaching out for contact, crying when in need but stopping when the need was satisfied. Roland managed all of these.

We worked on all the above stimulation exercises with Roland, and they produced positive results. In my view he was undoubtedly fortunate also to have a lively older sibling as a role model. Despite a wobbly right knee joint (displacing patella) which affects him to this day, Roland was walking at eleven months – only a month later than his older brother.

In fact, up to the age of 12 months, Roland more or less kept up with normal developmental milestones. Roland exhibited most of the behaviours expected of a child his age but was unusually slow in some responses, such as if the top of his head were gently touched in such a way that he couldn't see where the touch had come from, he would look puzzled for a moment then he would slowly move his hand towards the location of the touch rather than instantly registering its position. We noticed that Roland tended to acquire skills by imitation and memory rather than working things out for himself.

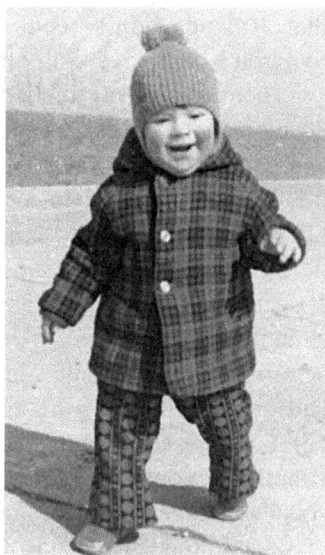

FIRST STEPS: 1977

Warren developed a close bond with him and never showed frustration with his younger brother's limitations.

Unlike some children with his condition, Roland's hearing and vision appeared fairly normal and he began to repeat basic words in his own fashion. For a while we called him "Roly" – which he rendered as "Ooly".

Although he didn't exhibit any repetitive behaviours, special aptitudes, fixations or obsessions at this age, Roland's food preferences were rather odd. He took a while to graduate from a milk and milky porridge diet and one stage would only consume evaporated milk and beef soup from tins. His next favourite was rather more balanced: home-made beef stew blended to break down lumps.

As it became clear that we were coping with Roland's basic needs and that he appeared to be thriving, attention from the NHS and ancillary services gradually fell away. Pat was content to do most of the routine child-care as I was in full-time employment. Although my job took me round the county, my office was local so I would often pop in at lunchtime and help with meals then top up my required hours by working on documents in the evening. I also supervised all Warren and Roland's street play.

Around Roland's second birthday we had a visit from an educational psychologist. This was to be expected in the light of Roland's condition. He put Roland through a series of tests to assess his levels of knowledge and comprehension. Roland scored quite well on recognition and naming of objects such as house, flower, plate etc. However, he struggled with numbers, and with speaking in sentences. Intriguingly, Roland scored more highly if Pat and I could see the pictures being pointed at – even though we were careful not to show any reaction to them. He retained this non-verbal communication ability. Provided topics being cogitated upon are not too abstract, Roland sometimes repeats word for word what I am thinking.

The psychologist's conclusion was that Roland clearly had learning difficulties and assessed his IQ in the range 50-60. IQ scores don't seem to be quoted so much nowadays but they do relate to mental ability. A graph of IQ against population has a bell-shape so the majority of people would score between 90 and 110 at the top of the bell curve. On both sides of the bell shape, the numbers in the population drop off steeply. People with IQs over 150 are quite rare and rate as highly gifted intellectually. Conversely people with IQs of 80 and below are also fairly uncommon, but they have significant learning difficulties. 50-60 IQ wasn't bad for a child with Downs but nevertheless meant that Roland would need special education – following a Statement of Special

Educational Needs. In those days, the classification was "educationally sub-normal – severe" or ESN(S). In addition to the usual child benefit, we were told about entitlement to Invalid Care Allowance – which subsequently morphed into Disability Living Allowance and much later was replaced by Personal Independence Payment, Employment Support Allowance and then Universal Credit. So, support processes were kick-started, and things got moving.

Any parent can ask for an educational assessment for their child if they consider there are special needs. In Roland's case, because of his Downs diagnosis shortly after birth, the assessment was done automatically.

So, at the tender age of two years, Roland found himself provided with a local special school placement. I don't remember much involvement by the social services once he was at school, although it's possible that social workers visited the school. The only feedbacks I recall were regular age-appropriate school reports and the occasional phone calls and letters about school events.

This would probably not be the case today. Apart from the downward pressure on educational budgets, the policy currently seems to be integration with mainstream provision, with ancillary help provided to deal with any additional issues such as sensory impairment, mobility, challenging behaviours etc.

In conversation with my dad – who was deputy head of a school for the physically handicapped – he remarked somewhat sardonically that children with Downs tended to become the "elite" of ESN(S) schools. Roland certainly fitted in straightaway at the Kettering special education unit. The staff were very kind and while there was transport, Pat sometimes found it more convenient to take Roland to school using the child seat on the back of her push-bike. The special school hours chimed fairly well with other domestic routines.

Roland's teacher, who had a few children with Downs in her class, introduced us to the term "Downs heap" – an uncooperative sitting position adopted by her pupils when they didn't want to get up or be picked up. It entailed relaxation of muscles already low in tone to the point where it was difficult to get a grip. The fairly common combination of reduced muscle tone with hyper-extensible joints also made it possible for these children to relax in poses that would otherwise be acutely uncomfortable. This certainly applied to Roland though he rarely went into Downs heap mode as he liked receiving attention and being picked up.

The school environment and its lesson structures meant that Roland was learning and practising new skills aimed at promoting self-help by imitation and repetition. Progress with toilet and personal hygiene training routines at home was slow and inconsistent. It was time-consuming and difficult to maintain with the other demands of family life. Thus, it became easier and more efficient to do it for him, but this set up behaviour patterns which much later took a long time and a lot of patient care to undo.

Going to his nursery school was key in providing Roland with ample opportunity to mix with other children and interact with adults outside the family circle. The concept of sharing and using simple social language such as "hello", "goodbye", "please" and "thank-you" was reinforced. This seemed to come quite easily to Roland as he was naturally sociable. However, he was, and is, a rather lazy communicator. Although he developed a fairly good vocabulary early on, as shown by his ability to name a wide variety of objects, and to understand and respond to what was said to him, he tended not to speak in sentences if he could get away with using just one or two key words. So, it was usually a waste of time to offer him two choices in one sentence. If he was in a positive mood, he would say yes to everything. If grumpy, there would be a series of "Nos". But if Roland was annoyed about something and felt he was not being listened to, he would put a sentence together that made his feelings quite clear! Conversely if he was shocked or hurt, he could become tongue-tied.

Neither Pat nor I were very sociably inclined so visitors to the house tended to be limited to close or extended family. Nevertheless, we agreed that it was important for both Warren and Roland to have the opportunity to mix with their peers and make friends. In Kettering we were fortunate to have Wicksteed Park nearby. It then had traditional playground equipment such as swings, slides, roundabouts and climbing frames but also a boating lake with a miniature railway running around it. Warren and Roland soon gained physical confidence and familiarity with other kids. The reactions of adults varied. Some would take one glance at Roland and look away, but others would be curious and try to be encouraging, telling us they had this or that relative with a disabled child and would relate a positive anecdote.

We lived hallway up a hill, so Patrick and the bigger kids used to weave their way down on skateboards. I made soapbox carts for Warren, and Roland had a pedal car in the shape of an AA break-down vehicle. This was a great way to integrate Roland into the local community of youngsters. They all knew he was "mongol" (a term in common use in those days) but his friendly demeanour led to acceptance.

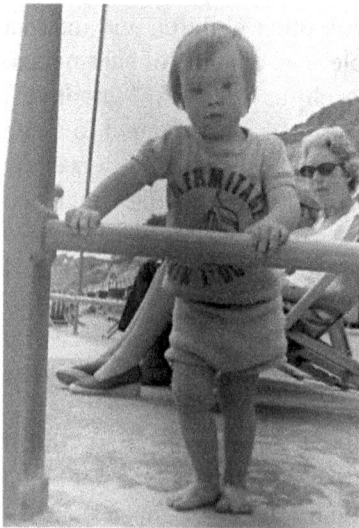

AT THE BEACH, 1979

He was adventurous in his simple way, not afraid to rattle down the hill in company with Warren. The only problem was that sometimes he would become distracted watching the scenery going by and run into an obstacle – usually a tree – whereupon he would start cursing the tree for getting in his way! I would tow Warren and Roland round the local streets. This caught on with the neighbours' kids and sometimes we would join several carts to make "trains" and hurtle down St Michael's Way with up to ten laughing and shouting kids on board. I wouldn't dare do it now – for fear of accidents – but luckily no-one ever got hurt. Later, Patrick won a cup at a soap box derby held at nearby Rockingham Castle. He became quite skilled at cycling and skateboarding, and later on he sailed through his motorcycle and car tests first time round.

In the 1970s camping wasn't as regulated as it is today, and a family could have inexpensive holidays this way if they had a tent and didn't mind roughing it. Roland was rather slow with his toilet training, so the guy ropes of our canvas ridge-tent were routinely festooned with towelling nappies strung along them like bunting. Otherwise, he adapted well to the primitive living conditions and was a good traveller – usually lulled to sleep by the droning vibration of our old cars. We had a folding twin pushchair which would comfortably hold Warren and Roland. They both enjoyed being wheeled around in this and it was a convenient way of carrying the clothes and provisions for days out at the beach. Our favourite places were Cromer in Norfolk, Weymouth in Dorset, and occasionally Blackpool and the Isle of Wight.

My brother John used to visit by train, as did James. Neither set of parents owned a car so we used to drive the 80 miles to London en famille and stay over for varying periods in the holidays. Pat's parents in particular enjoyed trips to the south coast where Roland developed an enduring fascination with theme parks. He enjoyed all the facilities: from the mildest tea-cup roundabouts to the most boisterous white-knuckle rides.

There was another member of the family, a seal-point Siamese cat. The name on his pedigree was Lecas Chantorm

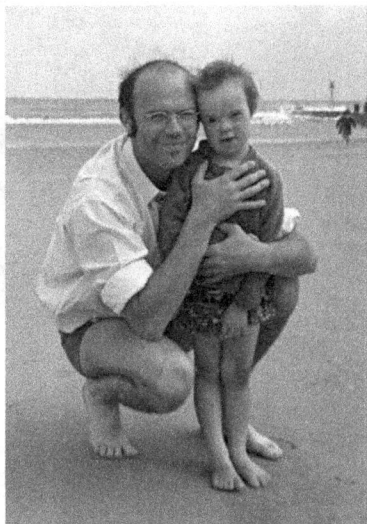

WITH DAD AT THE BEACH

but we renamed him Bruce after the martial artist whose films were popular in the 1970s and 1980s. As a young cat he was amazingly athletic. One of our neighbours had a dog which would yap annoyingly whenever we were in the back garden. One day Bruce leapt clean over the 4ft high brick wall dividing our gardens, landed squarely on the dog's back, boxed its ears and leapt back into our garden – all in a few seconds. The dog gave a yelp and ran indoors. It wasn't so noisy after that. Roland loved Bruce, and the cat was very patient with him – occasionally permitting Roland to use him as a pillow!

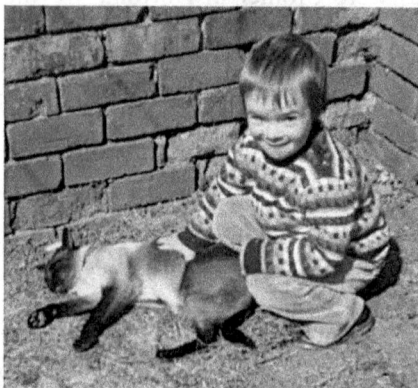

WITH BRUCE, THE SIAMESE CAT

3: Early Schooling –
Age 5 to 10 Years

Roland reaching mainstream school-age early in 1981 coincided with a workplace promotion for me and the family moving to Leicestershire. Patrick decided to remain in Northants with his wife-to-be. His future in-laws had offered the couple use of a disused bungalow on their poultry farm, and Patrick was earning a small wage as a trainee engineer, so at eighteen, he was keen to grow up and leave home. This simplified Pat's role in running the home – though she missed Patrick's company.

We bought an attractive though un-modernized cottage, but before we could organize a grant for such modern facilities as a damp proof course, modern wiring, an inside loo and central heating, there came the coldest winter I'd ever known. Washing would freeze to board-like hardness as it was hung out, and when we tried to clear a path to the outside loo by sprinkling salt on the sheet ice it would fracture with a loud cracking sound before giving up and melting. We ran an electric convector heater in the kids' bedroom through the freezing nights, but the five-year-old Roland didn't like the red indicator light. He thought it was an eye looking at him and kept switching the heater off!

Self-help books for parents recommended due diligence when assessing the standard of special education on offer from local authorities. The suggested approach included reviewing your child's Statement of Special Educational Needs, ascertaining your rights and expected roles as parents and asking several questions. For example: can you meet the teachers and have a look round the special school – or the unit attached to the mainstream school? If transport and ancillary support such as school medicals, speech therapy etc. has not already been offered, ascertain that the school is equipped to provide these services. Having done these preliminary checks, are you satisfied with what is being offered and that you will be involved in annual reviews?

We were again fortunate with Warren and Roland's schooling. They fitted in quickly and liked their teachers. Warren's school was within walking distance, but Roland's was quite a distance away in Loughborough. Fortunately, transport was provided and, due to the shorter school hours, Roland's new daily routine fitted in fairly well with Warren's.

From memory, Roland's brief schooldays at Loughborough were more about play and acquiring basic social skills than learning the "three Rs". But in terms of the expected learning stages like social, cognitive, physical/motor, language, self-help etc. he continued to do reasonably well. He enjoyed play, listening to music, and looking at simple books. Although running was difficult for him, Roland learned to swim and ride a bicycle with trainer wheels – though he wasn't very good at applying the brakes!

His toilet training remained fairly basic in that he wasn't very good at cleaning himself afterwards – so we always included spare underpants and trousers in his day-bag. We facilitated dressing and undressing by providing trousers with elasticated waistbands and shoes with Velcro fastenings. We paid for school lunches – which Roland seemed happy with despite his dislike of fresh vegetables – especially peas!

Ofsted was not formed until the early 1990s and, as far as I know, Roland's Statement of Special Educational Needs remained largely unchanged.

Roland had always been quite food-oriented and was developing a quirky sense of humour. When asked his name by strangers he would sometimes reply "Roland Egg" or "Roland Sausage". Following a school Bible-story lesson he was asked to recall who had performed the miracle of the loaves and fishes. "Jesus Crust" he replied.

An unexpected career opportunity entailed a family move to Farnborough, Hampshire only two years later in 1983. At least the house was in good order so we could move straight in. We were also much closer to London so we could visit our parents more often. Roland had received such positive reports from the Loughborough school that we were encouraged to put him forward for a place at an ESN(M) school when we moved – for pupils with only mild learning difficulties. This proved to be a mistake.

The school was in nearby Aldershot – a place dominated by army establishments. Roland went from being one of the most able and socially-adjusted in his class to near the bottom of a group of kids who were mostly just rather slow learners by normal standards. The class size was also larger compared to his first school, so Roland received less attention and encouragement.

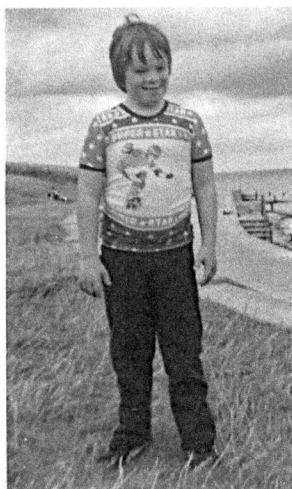

CHEEKY CHAPPIE

The result was that, in contrast to his normally equable demeanour, Roland reacted by being "lumpish" and uncooperative with occasional angry outbursts both in school and at home. We agreed that he should revert to an ESN(S) school in Farnborough, and in the more easy-going environment he immediately became less unsettled. He went on to enjoy skiing and tobogganing in Bulgaria on a school trip in 1984 - something that probably would not happen these days in terms of taking such young kids abroad without their parents.

Things at home were far from ideal. I had to commute to London, and I had longer working hours in my demanding new job at the

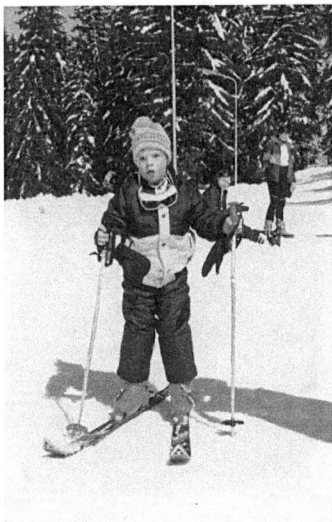

SKIING IN BULGARIA: 1984

Cabinet Office in Whitehall. Two moves in two years took their toll on family life, which is a balancing act for any family and relationship, especially with a special needs child in the mix. Pat was running the house virtually single-handedly, not only having to cope with a reactive and moody Roland but also his brother who was unsettled by leaving a school and a home where he had been happy. Warren began to acquire a reputation for disobedience at school.

In retrospect, Farnborough is where Roland began to put on weight, and it probably started with comfort-eating. An overstretched Pat overcompensated with treats - given that Roland was unhappy at school, and that food always put him in a better mood. We didn't consider the consequences. Neither Roland nor Warren flourished in this three-year phase, and the high stress levels for us all prompted another change.

4: Secondary and Further Education - Age 11 to 17

Our next, and final, house move was again work-related, but this time to we moved to Saltash in Southeast Cornwall, an area which Pat loved despite her unhappy previous married life in nearby Tideford. Warren was now old enough to go to secondary school, and Roland was eleven.

Both of them arrived with poor school reports from the Hampshire Education Authority. Warren had to put up with starting in the lower streams of his classes, but one of Roland's new teachers was so concerned at the possible disruption to her class that she visited us at home and tried to persuade Pat and me to place Roland somewhere else. We managed to reassure her that he'd been unfairly demonized. Roland was taught in a special unit attached to the Saltash comprehensive school. Typical of units designed to cater for children with severe learning difficulties, the emphasis was on caring and support. The atmosphere was pleasant, and the teachers were welcoming and friendly, while the educational content was there, albeit light-touch.

In this environment Roland's social skills continued to develop – permitting attendance at special-needs clubs and supervised participation in activities out in the community.

Likewise, his comprehension and communication skills improved, so he was increasingly able to understand what was said or asked of him and to give appropriate verbal responses. He was able to run simple errands within the protected environment. He acquired basic reading and writing skills such as signing his name. He learned to tell the time from a

Downs Children - the Story of Roland

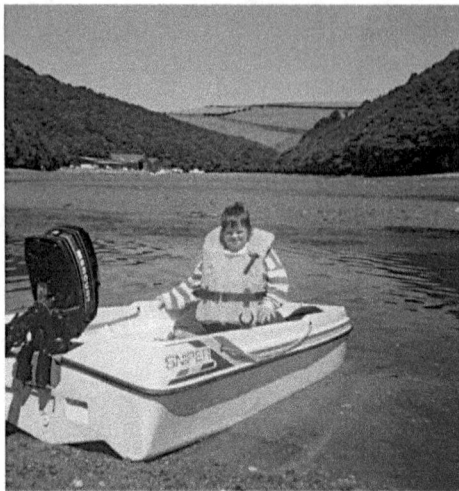

LOOE RIVER EXPEDITION: 1989

clock or watch and could recognize numbers up to twenty.

Roland always made sure he wore his digital watch. It seemed that, in addition to its obvious uses, the watch gave him a feeling of orientation and control. In particular he knew when to expect meals and when routine activities were due, such as getting up in the morning and when it was bed-time. He began to get a sense of longer time periods as indicated on a calendar, such as days of the week, forthcoming events and seasons of the year. It remained a mystery to him however that clocks went forward an hour in the spring and back again in autumn!

It became clear that, despite his limited cognitive abilities, Roland had a good concentration span and would steadily persist at tasks that interested him. Thus, he developed the ability to operate everyday domestic equipment such as radio, TV, DVD player, and a computer games console. He was careful with appliances - never breaking anything through clumsiness or impatience. He also became more adventurous and capable outside the home: riding a bike, swimming, using playground equipment such as swings, slides, climbing frames etc.

However, he did struggle with some things that might be considered routine. For example, managing personal hygiene effectively – especially after toileting. In the home he was nervous about handling hot objects, so he wasn't competent at cooking a basic meal and using a microwave, hob or oven. Likewise, using a washing machine, vacuum cleaner and doing other routine household tasks appeared to be beyond him at that age. Outside the home he obviously continued to need safeguarding, but even with support, handling money remained a puzzle to him – which impacted on his use of amenities, and participation in trips and holidays.

The varied abilities and personalities of his fellow Downs pupils and others in the special education unit belied any assumption that learning difficulties entailed individual uniformity. One Downs lad

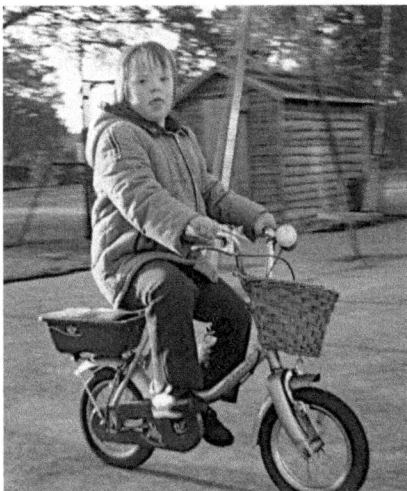

CYCLING: 1986

was tall and physically robust but his speech was impaired. Another was small in stature, wore spectacles and was partially deaf but encouraged by his parents, he went out and about in the local community on his own. Yet another had near-normal conversational and other skills despite having very marked Downs' facial features.

Downs girls seemed a little quicker to learn than the boys and they tended to be mischievous and flirtatious. The latter trait was likely to be a concern for parents and carers when their daughters reached child-bearing age.

An attempt was made to integrate Roland and some of his classmates into a mainstream class but although he could rub along with the other first year boys and girls, the lesson content was too demanding for him, so the experiment was discontinued after one term. Instead, Roland attended classes at Saltash College and another special education unit attached to Plymouth College of Further Education. Transport was provided via a local taxi firm.

Roland enjoyed the varied classes which concentrated on practical topics: domestic science, reading and writing and simple math, recognizing money, self-advocacy etc. He was popular with his teachers at both units as he had a good memory, he could concentrate for fairly long periods, and he was well-behaved. Indeed, he was sometimes put next to the more restless or scatter-brained students because he was generally tolerant and had a calming effect on them. One of the teaching assistants at Saltash College invited Roland to an evening club for learning-disabled youngsters held at a local church hall. Fortnightly attendance at Tamar Friends, as it was later called, became a social experience for Roland that he really enjoyed.

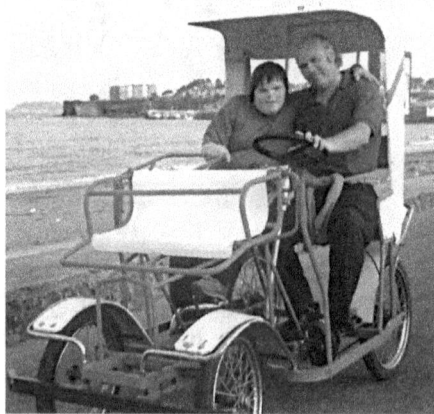

ON FOUR WHEELS: 1993

It was during our early years in Saltash that the teenage Roland had two potentially disastrous mishaps. They occurred during visits to London when we were staying with Pat's parents and Pat's younger brother James.

Roland loved travelling on the London Underground and as I had some shopping to do in the city, I took Warren and Roland with me. All went well until it was time for Roland to get off the train. He grumbled and whinged and dragged his feet, insisting on lagging behind once we exited at street level. I was intent on completing my shopping trip and pressed on, turning at intervals to make sure Roland was following. Suddenly I lost sight of him in the crowd of pedestrians. Warren and I hurried back but Roland was nowhere to be seen – though I thought I'd heard him shout. Suppressing a feeling of panic, I reported the situation to a policeman who called in Roland's description. After casting about fruitlessly for another half hour I took Warren to my in-laws' place wondering helplessly if Roland was all right. James opened the door, and his first words were "He's been found!" A policeman had called round and said Roland was safe and well.

He'd been spotted wandering in and out of shops and been taken to a police station and Pat was en route to collect him. When he returned, Roland seemed no worse for his experience. He was clutching a police pamphlet which had been signed by all the officers at the station. Possibly because they knew how contrary and balky Roland could be, no-one blamed me – though I blamed myself.

The second drama happened during a walk in a country park with Pat and Warren. Roland had started complaining that he wanted to go home. On the way back to the car we walked through some woodland in which there was a wide drainage ditch, its water surface covered with pondweed. We had crossed this using a bridge then emerged into an open field, but Roland, who was deliberately keeping his distance, failed to appear. We were on the point of retracing our steps when he came into view. His gait looked rather odd, but it wasn't until he drew closer that we saw he was soaked and covered from head to toe in pondweed. "Green!" he exclaimed, picking at the weed adhering to his face and hair. We concluded that he had tried to walk across the ditch (the weed-covered surface of which did look rather like a carpet) instead of using the bridge – and had become submerged. Somehow, he had scrambled out under his own power. This episode, which was comical at the time, could so easily have ended in tragedy. Roland's ability to swim had evidently stopped him from panicking and this had saved his life.

Adolescence certainly also brought a certain feistiness to Roland's demeanour – no doubt influenced by his older brother. They provoked each other in a fraternal manner and Roland acquired a vocabulary of swear-words with somewhat alarming ease. Although Warren was more than a match for Roland in every respect, Roland could hold his own in rough and tumbles because he had a surprising degree of upper body strength. On one occasion Roland aimed an uppercut, but Warren saw it coming and blocked with both arms. Nevertheless, the impact momentarily lifted Warren's feet clear of the floor.

Regarding girls, Roland liked them and would offer hugs accompanied by goofy grins, but there was no overtly sexualized behaviour. Girls tended to like him too. They regarded him as cuddly both in build and temperament – and thus relatively harmless.

There was a Boy Scout hut in the service lane bordering the end of our back garden and Roland was invited to take part in some of their activities. His unstable right knee joint and increasing weight stopped him from running but he was good at games where he had to hold a line and prevent other boys from forcing their way through. He gained a reputation for being "hard" though it should be said that all his Scout mates were younger than him.

Medically, Roland continued to be generally healthy. However, his increasing weight was becoming an issue and he suffered from time to time with urinary tract infections and he also had a suspected epileptic seizure. This occurred after we had bought him a larger TV to go with his computer games console, so the brightness and flickering of the new screen (pre-LED days) may have triggered the attack. He underwent tests at Treliske Hospital in Truro, but the results were inconclusive. Nevertheless, from then on, we made sure he had dark glasses to wear if he went to discos or other venues where there was flashing or strobe lighting.

5: Adult Social Care/Day Centres and Clubs - Age 18 Plus

Prior to our move to Cornwall, Social Services involvement had been minimal. Occasionally a social worker would turn up, ask how we were doing, offer helpful advice on state benefits and other support available, then leave us to get on with life. However, once Roland was past school leaving age, Cornwall Council Adult Social Care assumed a degree of legal responsibility for Roland's welfare and support. Care plans were drawn up and Roland's needs were assessed as "substantial" which meant he was eligible for day services mostly funded by the local authority. Pat was designated Roland's main carer, and he was allocated a case co-ordinator who reported to a qualified social worker. From time to time, it was suggested that it would be in Roland's best interests to leave home and go into supported living. But Pat couldn't bear the idea of "losing

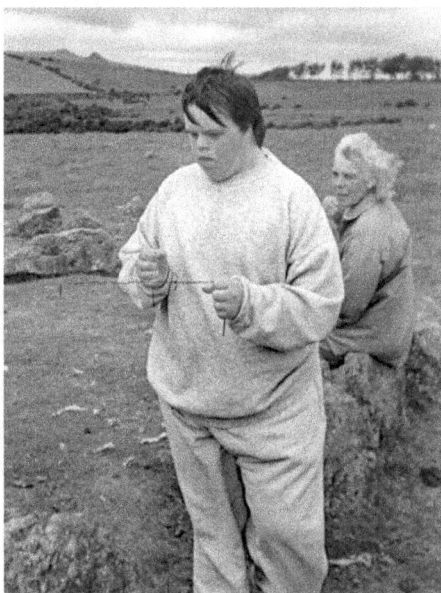

DOWSING ON DARTMOOR: 1994

him" so I didn't press the point – though the concept made sense to me.

A place was found for Roland at Morley Tamblyn Lodge – a council-owned day centre fourteen miles away at Liskeard. This placement followed another assessment of his needs by Adult Social Care, and the free package included transport to and from Morley Tamblyn Lodge by minibus. Roland's social skills meant that he fitted in well with the other service users – several of whom he knew from his school and college placements. In addition to arts and crafts, gardening, drama and simple computer work, activities included supervised trips using minibus and public transport. Despite his continued progress in various areas, it was clear that Roland was not ready for paid or volunteer work at home or outside or living away from the parental home.

It wasn't that Roland was incapable of the activities listed above, it was more a matter of the training he was receiving outside the home not being practised and consolidated at home. Pat didn't expect Roland ever to grow up – and perhaps she didn't want him to. To her he was a like an oversized baby, with a free lifetime subscription to "Hotel Mama". My attempts to persuade her that it would be in Roland's best interests to practise as many independence skills as possible were rebuffed. Worse, the subject of Roland's diet was a "hot potato". He was getting fatter for reasons that were unclear inasmuch that we were all eating much the same and not becoming obese, but Pat became so upset when I suggested putting Roland on a reducing diet that the effort was counter-productive.

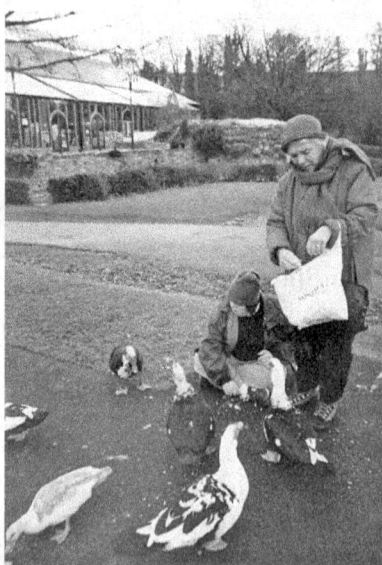

FEEDING BIRDS WITH MUM: 1995

The decade 1990-2000 took its toll on all of us. Between 1990 and 1995 both Pat's parents and my father all died after short illnesses. Pat's younger brother James, who'd had to give up a theology degree course in his twenties due to developing a mental illness, was left alone in his London home and needed a lot of support. Psychiatric social workers supplied most of this, but I took responsibility for his finances and visited him in London regularly. In 1995, still traumatized by the loss of my Dad, my Mum sold up in London and came to live nearby and she also needed a lot of emotional and practical support.

In 1998 William's marriage to Lou broke up and he came to visit us from Germany with their two young children. On his return journey he nearly died in a freak car accident. Miraculously the two kids were unhurt and their mum, Lou, arrived from Germany to take care of them. For two months Pat and I were frequent visitors to Bristol Infirmary where William slowly recovered from his injuries. But after he returned overseas a bitter divorce battle began and Pat took Lou's side – distancing herself from William.

I qualified in therapeutic massage and aromatherapy and practised at a local complementary therapy centre in Plymouth in my spare time. Roland enjoyed trying out a range of physical therapies at open days and local festivals.

Also, in 1998 Roland had a circumcision under general anaesthetic to improve urine flow, as he was increasingly prone to urinary tract infections (UTIs). He coped with the anaesthesia well and the operation gave him some relief from the problem for several years.

6: Looking towards the Future - Age 24 to 34 (2000 - 2010)

Advice from the Downs Childrens Association and other sources told us that Pat and I should make wills that included special provision for Roland. Although we would have wanted to make such provision anyway, there were stories about parents who cut their disabled offspring out of their wills on the assumption that the state would provide for them. Apart from the questionable probity of this approach we were advised that such inequitable wills were open to legal challenge by the local authority, who were otherwise likely to be saddled with the full cost of care after parents had passed away. Costly legal wrangles could go on for years and deplete whatever funds had been inherited.

The recommended procedure was to set up a Discretionary Trust in favour of the disabled person and to will an equitable proportion of the estate to the Trust. This meant that the disabled person's entitlement to state benefits was not reduced. The MENCAP charity was also recommended as an administrator of such arrangements. In addition, MENCAP offered a visiting service whereby independent inspectors would regularly visit the home of the disabled person to check that they were being well-treated, that the wishes of the Trustees were being complied with, and to take action if not. There would be fees for these services.

In connection with the above, it was also considered sensible to set up lasting powers of attorney (LPAs) so that parents and/or carers had the authority to make decisions on behalf of disabled persons who had limited capacity to manage their own affairs. Pat and I made appropriate wills and set up a discretionary trust with the assistance of a solicitor, but we deferred action on LPAs.

At the end of 2005, I took early retirement to support Pat in the care of Roland as her energy levels and stamina were noticeably declining. At the time I put this down to her age but with hindsight I now link it with the slow onset of dementia.

My mum's situation was also a factor. By now she had been living in her Saltash bungalow for ten years and she was happy there. She was a regular visitor for meals, games of Scrabble and walks in the local countryside. However, she was slowly losing her central vision due to macular degeneration, and at 85 years of age, she needed more support and reassurance. It dawned on me that I might find myself the sole carer for three people.

By this time Roland had become grossly overweight. He was only 5 feet 2 inches tall but weighed 19 stone.

Walking quickly tired him so we got used to taking a wheelchair with us on outings. Mags, a therapeutic colleague, used to visit and give Roland "Indian head" massages. Mags seemed to enjoy giving Roland these treatments as much as he enjoyed receiving them. She would engage him in conversation and was amused by the way he relaxed so quickly – often so completely that he fell asleep. Mags noticed that we had a traditional African goat-skinned drum (djembe), and suggested Roland might enjoy attending Africussion – a Plymouth-based group that welcomed drummers at all ability levels.

In August 2006 Pat and I attended a performance of Oklahoma at the Sterts open air theatre, Upton Cross, Cornwall. A local actress had masterminded a project to involve learning disabled people in public performances. This led to Roland being given a bit part as a cowboy in the crowd

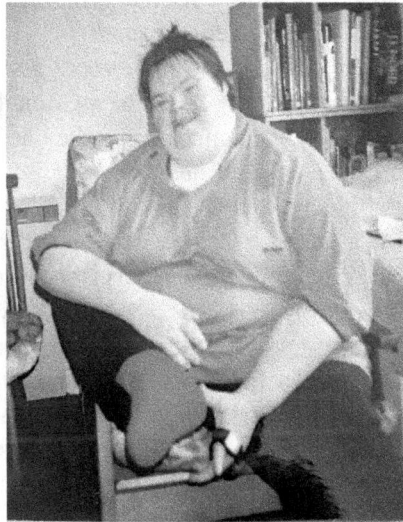

ROLAND WHEN OBESE: 2006

scenes – at one point being brought centre stage. He was also allowed to play his "baran" drum in support of the orchestra.

Later in the same month Pat and I saw "Return to the Forbidden Planet" also at Sterts Theatre. Roland again played his drum with the band. His appearances, along with other service users from his day centres, were a result of the continuing engagement of his drama teacher with local professional groups.

Roland also enjoyed going to the Quest Festivals held at Newton Abbot racecourse. These offered lots of New Age and folk music, together with opportunities to sample a variety of therapies.

2006 also saw my first meeting with retired teacher and community worker, Tilly, at a local complementary health centre. Like me, she had an interest in astrology and she joined the local group meetings. She also met Roland when I took him to the socials.

Tilly moved from Plymouth to Landrake – three miles from Saltash. Unbeknown to me she had befriended my mum Polly, along with one of my mum's elderly acquaintances who lived in Landrake and who used to attend the Methodist Church there. Tilly was to play a major role in my family's future as she and Polly became very close.

In 2008, Pat and I attended a meeting at Morley Tamblyn Lodge (MTL) – Roland's Council-run day centre - with his social worker and key-worker at the centre. Roland was also present as the meeting was to discuss his future. It was established that Roland was happy with his current activities at MTL and at a local workshop and smallholding called The Craft Barn – and that his supervisors were happy with him. However, his obesity was an issue, and it was agreed a Learning Disability Nurse should see him and carry out tests for thyroid deficiency and diabetes, and maybe offer dietary advice. There was also a discussion about a future residential placement, but no firm conclusion was reached – though apparently it was possible for a person to come out of such a placement if they weren't happy, without jeopardizing subsequent applications. It was suggested that Roland could have a trainer allocated for a couple of hours per week to get him out and about, and that there might be other daytime activities available.

In December of that year Pat and I went to the MTL production of Cinderella. Roland and a friend played ugly sisters, though in a break with tradition the friend wore a suit and was called George. Drama teacher Sue produced and directed the panto and stayed on stage throughout, keeping up the momentum. Roland looked the part in a green dress with a fur stole – but one of the high (or maybe low) spots in the show occurred when the other ugly sister's trousers fell down in the middle of a speech and he made no attempt to cover himself.

2009 and 2010 passed with Roland continuing to enjoy his day-centre events, which included drama productions, barbecues and a barn dance. He also joined the monthly drumming workshop that Mags had told us about.

Annual medical checks showed he remained generally healthy apart from being obese.

In December 2010 Roland's new social worker Nathan and female trainee Lettie made a home visit to carry out an assessment on Roland. Nathan patiently went through a long questionnaire gathering information about Roland's home life, activities, medical issues, likes and dislikes etc. He was particularly intrigued about Roland's habit of sleeping in the lounge with the light and TV on all night - and he was concerned about his sedentary lifestyle and weight - though he acknowledged efforts were being made with Roland's diet and outside activities. Nathan's conclusion was that Roland's needs remained graded as "substantial" and that he would recommend a further assessment by the Learning Disability team with a view to reviewing his diet and a possible exercise regime.

The end of 2010 also saw my mother, Polly's, decision to leave her bungalow and move into a local care home at the age of ninety. Failing eyesight and unreliable short-term memory were making independent life difficult, despite support from Tilly and me. Also, Pat was beginning to distance herself from Polly and other family members – saying she no longer enjoyed having regular visitors. I took over more household tasks, particularly driving, as Pat was losing her confidence.

Downs Children - the Story of Roland

Early in 2011, there was a Person-Centred Planning (PCP) meeting organized by Adult Social Care. I took Roland along. It emerged that additional money might be made available for day activities. The interview consisted mainly of listing Roland's likes and dislikes. One of the exercises involved Roland drawing a series of concentric circles and marking within them the people important to him – with the most important in the inmost circle, then outwards in decreasing order. Remarkably considering his brief acquaintance, Roland put Tilly's name in an inner circle along with other close family members. He ranked likes and dislikes in a similar manner.

His pal Rufus was there with his Mum. She seemed to think the process was poorly organized and relied too much on an expectation that learning-disabled people would be able to articulate their needs effectively. I was inclined to agree but said I would attend the next session.

In April I took Roland to see a podiatrist at Liskeard Community Hospital, and the podiatrist fitted insoles into his shoes as a gentle corrective to the congenital mis-alignment of his knees and ankles. No further appointments were considered necessary.

In May, a second PCP meeting took place in Saltash. Having completed a list of Roland's family members and friends – plus a list of likes and dislikes - at the previous meeting, we were encouraged to list his various activities in order of preference. I spent some time talking to Kylie, who explained that at Roland's next assessment there would probably be discussion of his personal budget. Kylie said that only people with needs classed as substantial or critical would be offered a Personal Budget (PB). It would then be up to the disabled person and carers to research suitable activities and pay for them out of the budget. Apparently, Cornwall Council had been very slow implementing this and now they were rolling out the scheme at a time of major budget cuts. Theoretically service-users could opt to continue at the council-owned Morley Tamblyn Lodge (MTL) but the cynic in me wondered if the hidden agenda was to erode usage of the Centre so it could be closed down and sold off. One potentially useful point raised by Kylie was the possibility of a free pass to the Saltash Leisure Centre. This reminded me of the letter written to our family GP in February 2011 by Zelda (a physio at Liskeard) about getting Roland some supervised gym training. I therefore reminded the surgery of this letter and they said we would be sent a form.

At the end of May I took Roland to join with his drumming group in support of the Plymouth half-marathon. Having parked near the Moat House Hotel with the benefit of Roland's disabled parking badge, I wheeled Roland in his chair to the Hoe near the top of Elliott Street and linked up with drum tutor Jon, his partner Mary, and some other drummers who were clustered round Jon's VW Camper sipping tea and eating carrot cake. The weather was cool, and the sky was overcast with the occasional hint of misty rain – good running conditions but not so great for goatskin drums. The first runners had already passed before we assembled and started to play. Roland had his small lightweight drum with mylar skin, and I played my recently purchased "festival djembe" which also featured a man-made skin. These two drums were not only light to carry, but their skins maintained tension in the damp air unlike traditional goat-skinned djembes. We drummed for nearly two hours until the last of the competitors had passed by. There were appreciative waves from the runners, and we were photographed several times. At the end, Jon said he was pleased with the session, and we returned to his van for another cup of tea before dispersing.

Later that month, I took Pat and Roland on a boat trip to Calstock organized by an out and about group. This had been formed by parents of children with learning difficulties, and Roland had recently been invited to join. Its founder member Una was an effective activist who continually pressed Adult Social Care to live up to its responsibilities. The calm, fine weather was ideal for a river trip, and everyone enjoyed it. There was time for a pasty lunch at Calstock before the return journey. The trip took just over an hour each way. At three in the afternoon of the same day, I took Roland for his annual medical check-up. His blood pressure was satisfactory at 138/88, but his weight had increased to 19stone 7lbs. The nurse said she would chase our GP regarding the supervised gym sessions suggested by physio Zelda – as he had not responded to a letter and reminder. We were about to leave when another nurse bustled in and requested a blood sample for thyroid testing. Roland wasn't happy but he endured the procedure – despite his dislike of needles.

In September, Roland enjoyed a couple of events at the Saltash Football Clubhouse with the out and about group, including a disco arranged at the Saltash Football Club and a pizza and samba evening. They were impressed when he played the drums.

Pat and I delivered Roland to MTL on the afternoon of Friday 30th for his sleepover camp and Saturday day-trip to Looe. His eight fellow campers and the staff were in excellent spirits due to the unseasonably warm and sunny weather. They dropped him off at the Saltash Wesley Church on Saturday evening. Everyone seemed to have had a good time – though Roland was rather quiet after the event, and he slept solidly for ten hours after returning home.

Early in October 2011, Pat slipped and fell on the rockery near the top of the back garden. I was mowing the grass at the time, so I didn't see it happen. But on switching the mower off I heard her call and found her nursing her left forearm which had apparently borne the brunt of the fall. I lifted her to her feet and helped her to a chair. There wasn't much to see but the wrist was swelling, and it was clearly very tender. At the suggestion of the Medical Centre, we went to St Barnabas Hospital in Saltash who examined the arm and in turn referred us to the Cumberland Centre in Plymouth. There X-rays revealed a crack in the distal end of the radius – near the wrist. A temporary cast was applied, and an appointment made for the Derriford Fracture Clinic the following Wednesday. At the Fracture Clinic, we saw a consultant orthopaedic surgeon who said that the fracture went right through the bone, which was displaced. He recommended an operation under general anaesthetic to fix it in correct alignment using a titanium plate and screws, and with some trepidation Pat agreed to this.

The procedure was carried out on the twelfth of October, and Pat was kept in overnight. When I went to collect her from Derriford, the nursing staff were initially doubtful if she was fit to be discharged as she seemed vague and disoriented - but they eventually released her into my care. Over the next few days, she perked up, but her level of alertness did not seem fully to recover.

In conversation with the mother of one of Roland's friends about local residential units for people with learning difficulties, she said there were three such in Saltash to her knowledge – all run by the same company.

A couple of days later, it became obvious that Roland was suffering with his right big toe, so I took him to the doctor. He immediately diagnosed an infection in Roland's toe and prescribed Flucloxacillin. He thought the infection may have got into the toe by the ingrowing toenail, but he stopped short of recommending the removal of the nail.

As Roland's right big toe was still troubling him a week later, we returned to the Medical Centre and this time, we saw a different doctor. He thought that gout was also a possibility, so Roland was prescribed more Flucloxacillin plus Indometacin. This marked the end of Roland's second week of absence from day centres due to his walking difficulties.

Roland eventually returned to MTL and The Craft Barn smallholding for the last week before Christmas, after a month's break due to his infected right foot. Though walking was still uncomfortable, he enjoyed seeing his friends and distributing the Christmas cards he had spent hours writing out, and of course, he received cards and gifts in return.

In January 2012, the Social Services case co-ordinator, Lesley, came to interview the three of us at home. The purpose was to begin the process of assessing Roland for a personal budget. She also arranged a meeting at MTL to review Roland's day activities.

At the end of that month Pat and I went to a review meeting at MTL. Liz had been appointed Roland's keyworker. Teri – the new manager of MTL – introduced herself and Lesley was also present. The meeting revolved around Roland's day activities. We finished with quite a long list of things that he liked to do and might benefit from. I suggested it would be good to factor some gentle exercise into his day placements – whilst emphasizing his proneness to injury from falls.

In February, Lesley visited us at home to complete a risk-assessment questionnaire as part two of the personal budget assessment process. Pat also completed a carer's self-assessment questionnaire. By careful questioning, Lesley established that the cause of Roland's bruised right elbow – which had effectively been denying him the use of his right arm over the last week – was him slipping on the wet floor of The Craft Barn crib-hut and banging his arm on the table.

I took Roland to the medical centre for his sore elbow and a suspected urinary tract infection (he was wetting his trousers and his urine looked cloudy). The doctor said the elbow was just bruised and would get better on its own. However, he prescribed Trimethoprim for the peeing issues.

Lesley visited for her third interview with us and with Roland as part of his personal budget setting process. This meeting was supposed to be brief and concerned only with ascertaining Roland's ability to handle money. It soon became evident that his recognition of currency was good, but he was uncertain about counting up different denominations and unsure how to work out change. Lesley went on to review her findings and fill in gaps. Inter alia she suggested Roland should have his eyes tested – as this had not been done for many years.

Following the suggestion by Lesley, I took Roland for an eye test at the new Specsavers place in Saltash where Pat had recently been prescribed her driving and reading glasses. The newly qualified optician took Roland through the standard tests and concluded that he had a "lazy" right eye which his brain tended not to use unless the left eye was covered up. Thus, although the vision of the right eye could be improved by the use of lenses, this would have no practical effect since the left eye was dominant and provided adequate vision. Both eyes were otherwise healthy. There was no prescription for spectacles.

Lesley visited to carry out her last interview with us regarding assessment of Roland for a personal budget. Roland was under the weather with a chesty cough, but he put in an appearance. The interview and form-filling seemed to go well, and Lesley said it would be a few weeks before we heard how much, if anything, Roland would be awarded. I quizzed her about an email comment by the "out and about" group leader, Una, that the more carers said they did for a claimant, the lower the budget would be. She confirmed this was so, adding that if we were to say we were unable to look after Roland he would get a large budget, but that his care would probably be taken out of our hands. It was a matter of balance – though Lesley also commented that so far none of her clients had ended up with less provision than they were getting before.

At the end of April, a continence nurse visited to see Roland in response to Lesley's recommendation. The interview was positive in tone, but the only recommendation was that Roland should try wearing pants with integral dribble pads to reduce "turnover" of trousers.

Lesley visited to put the finishing touches to Roland's personal budget and support plan. She confirmed he could have an extra day at MTL. Roland plumped for doing ten-pin bowling at St Austell on Fridays. It was also agreed that he could have a personal trainer for two hours each Saturday who would take him to the local gym.

In July, occupational therapist Connie visited to assess Roland's needs regarding toileting, washing and use of stairs. Various options were discussed, but it was finally agreed that Social Services would fit a handrail down the length of the main staircase – and outside the front door. Later the same day, Roland's fitness training assistant, Ollie, visited and introduced himself. A Jamaican by birth – and looking much younger than his 55 years – he was full of enthusiasm for his role. We went to the local gym and an assistant patiently introduced Roland (and Ollie) to a walking machine and rowing machine. Roland was nervous of the walking machine and found it difficult to adjust his stride – but was happier on the rowing machine. Ollie felt the experience wouldn't be complete for Roland without a shower, so he went through this process. Overall, Roland seemed to find his introduction to the gym a positive experience – encouraged in no small measure by Ollie's can-do attitude.

7: Adulthood

On the eve of his 36th birthday, Roland's right knee gave way as he was walking to the car at The Craft Barn. Luckily, he wasn't hurt badly but the incident shook him. Later in the week I took Roland to the doctor regarding his recurring spots and sweat rash. The doctor dismissed suggestions from Lesley and Ollie that Diprobase would help and said that our ongoing treatments using Conotrane cream (similar to zinc and castor oil) were doing a "fantastic job". He issued a repeat prescription for Conotrane and a one-off for Daktacort (an anti-bacterial cream).

At the beginning of September 2012, Ollie and physio, Zelda, made a home visit to discuss introducing aquarobics into Roland's exercise routine. We all sat in the garden wearing straw hats and quaffing soft drinks in the warm sunshine. Zelda kindly offered to demonstrate the exercises at Saltash Leisure Centre in October.

Lesley visited to audit Roland's personal budget records. She was happy with these and later confirmed that any surplus money could be used to subsidize Tamar Friends, the drumming club and out-and-about events.

Zelda turned up as promised and she led Roland through some simple exercises to get him used to the water. You could see the delight on Roland's face when he realized the buoyancy of the water was allowing him to do knee-bends, and standing on one leg, which would normally be difficult or risky for him. Zelda was concerned that Roland might become over-tired, but he didn't want the session to end. During a five-minute break he spontaneously started swimming with his slow, effortless front crawl/doggy paddle stroke. Zelda was surprised but she didn't try to stop him. She swam with Roland to the deep end and back. Zelda said she hoped to have one more swim session with Roland in November, which Ollie should be able to attend.

She wanted to observe a gym session to see if there was any advice she could offer.

We took full advantage of the social and recreational activities available to Roland locally. These included musical events and pantos, day trips with his youth groups, drama productions at his day centres, pub meals and the like.

In May 2013, there was a disco boat trip on the Tamar with the out-and-about group. Pat decided to come along, and she surprised me by sitting next to a loudspeaker during most of the three-hour trip. It was too loud for me, so I alternated between the cold and breezy top deck with its picturesque views of the passing countryside – and the noisy lower deck crowded with dancers. Roland enjoyed it despite two rather messy toilet interludes, and he did justice to the buffet provided. A couple of the women asked him to dance. In the early evening of the same day, I took Roland to Rowlands travelling fair at Warfelton Field, Saltash. Roland went for a walk round the fairground, but the queues were long, and he was tired, so he only had one go on the ghost-train before returning home.

Warren invited us to a barbecue at his place in Somerset. The food was ready around 2.30 – way past Roland's usual lunchtime – but he waited patiently in the sunshine watching all the goings-on. The barbecue was excellent – a mix of chicken, lamb, sausage and beefburgers with plenty of salad. We took our time over the meal, and it was 4.30 before we finished eating.

In June, Roland had an NHS dental appointment at Saltash Medical Centre, and apart from having some tartar scraped from between his front teeth all was well.

Trouble arose at MTL when a complaint was made that the service users were not being adequately safeguarded. The complaint was anonymous, but it named several members of staff who were suspended from duty by their Council employers. Parents and carers were up in arms because as far as they were concerned, there was nothing wrong with the standards of care at MTL. Some of us were interviewed on local TV.

The investigation dragged on for weeks, and MTL ran at much reduced capacity with a skeleton staff. During this time Roland was offered alternative day-centre provision at The Gentian Centre, a privately run centre in Liskeard. This service was well-staffed and offered a variety of activities and he soon made new friends.

So, Roland was now attending three different council-funded day centres: MTL, The Craft Barn and The Gentian Centre, plus a monthly drumming club and the out-and-about group as well as Tamar Friends. Pat and I had one weekend per month respite – when Roland went to a hostel paid for by Adult Social Care. At home, he spent lots of time with his PlayStation and watching TV and videos, plus playing a wide variety of music CDs. At his day centres he continued to enjoy socializing and drama classes.

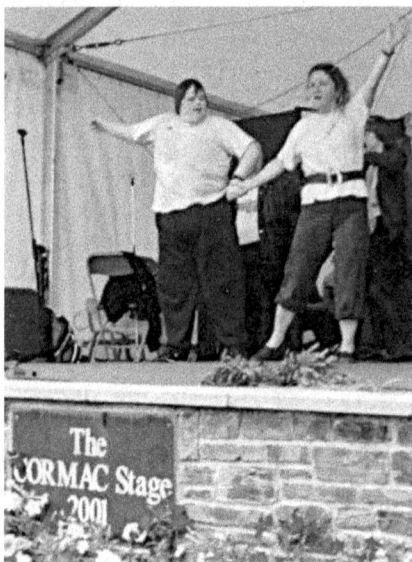

CORNWALL SHOW WITH SUE: 2012

At length, the MTL investigation came to an end, and it transpired that a disgruntled ex-employee had made the allegations. The suspended staff returned to work. By this time Roland was enjoying his Gentian Centre sessions but he wanted to return to MTL on Thursdays only – when he could do drama in the morning and help with producing the centre's newsletter in the afternoon.

Kit from The Gentian Centre rang to say how much they enjoyed having Roland on Tuesdays and Fridays. He added that although the Gentian Centre's daily rate was £6 higher than MTL's and the return trip by car/minibus was £20 per day, The Gentian Centre's staffing ratio was much higher than MTL's. I agreed that Roland seemed to like The Gentian Centre – but that we were waiting for news from Adult Social Care about Roland's options.

Later in the month, a meeting was convened at MTL by Adult Social Care to address ongoing grumbles from parents and carers.

The meeting was chaired by a senior manager and a woman from the Cornwall Council "cabinet". Managers from other day services and two independent facilitators were also present. The chairman endured barracking and interruptions but confirmed that all the suspended staff had been re-instated without adverse notes on their records and that recruitment of additional permanent staff was underway. He also said that MTL would re-open fully in August. In response to requests from parents and carers, chairman Pete agreed that there should be a steering group set up consisting of a councillor, officials from adult social care and parents/carers.

I asked if service users would be offered a choice of day centre provision if, like Roland, they had enjoyed the alternative provision while MTL was under-strength. The answer was yes. I took the opportunity to ask Pete if there was any truth in the rumour that the Council was considering putting the management of MTL out to contract and he replied that this idea was at a very early stage of consideration. Appointment of a new MTL manager, Mary, was confirmed. She undertook to look into concerns about poor security at MTL reception, difficulty in contacting reception by phone and erratic or absent catering facilities on site. The meeting ended with upbeat statements from the facilitators about the need to improve communications, cut out unnecessary bureaucracy and re-build trust at all levels.

At the end of the month, Bertha from Adult Social Care rang and agreed that Roland could return to MTL on Thursdays and have Tuesdays and Fridays at The Gentian Centre until further notice. The Craft Barn would be on Wednesdays only. I informed The Gentian Centre, The Craft Barn and MTL, and reminded Bertha that Pat and I would welcome more respite days.

In mid-August Pat, Roland and I went to see the national firework competition at Plymouth Hoe – viewed from a boat organized by the out and about group. The displays did not start till 9.30pm but we had to be at the Barbican by 5.30pm to get a place in the Elphinstone car park which offered level access to Commercial Wharf – where the Plymouth Princess tour-boat was waiting.

Roland embarked without too much difficulty and to kill time before the displays we spent from 7.30pm to 9.15pm on a mini-cruise to the Tamar Bridges and back which was very pleasant and scenic in the still, balmy air and smooth water. On our return, the captain made fast to a buoy less than ten metres from the Mountbatten Pier where the fireworks were arrayed, and we settled down to watch. All the displays were impressive. The concussions when the big star-shells burst had a visceral impact and the echoes from the Citadel walls were thunderous. The show finished on time, but it took until nearly midnight for us to get back to Saltash through long queues of traffic in the City Centre.

Later that month, Roland returned from a trip with The Gentian Centre to St Mellion golf club limping heavily and with a painful left ankle. It was unclear what had happened. It wasn't the first time a day-centre mishap had been inadequately explained – possibly in the hope of avoiding awkward questions from parents.

The following day a local stargazers and earth-mysteries group organized a trip to Soussons stone circle on Dartmoor. The day started inauspiciously with Roland unable to walk and having peed his bed and a few pairs of pyjamas. Fortunately, Pat and I had risen earlier than usual and were ready on time. We drove to nearby Landrake and picked Tilly up from her home. She backed Pat's view that we should take the wheelchair for Roland. By removing a crate of bits and pieces, we made room for the wheelchair. We went to Plymouth and picked up two more people en route to Dartmoor.

Roland was manoeuvred to the centre of the circle of stones in his wheelchair and oriented north/south. As we did so a breeze blew through the circle – the air had been still up to that point – then disappeared as suddenly as it had come. Afterwards some people reported seeing "power animals". One of my sensations was that something was sweeping across the landscape towards us from the south-west – then there was a brief impression of a crowd of hooded figures busying themselves near the circle. After a while spent vibe-sensing and dowsing for earth-energies, the group split up and went for pub lunches before re-convening at a historic church where there were relics of interest. Tilly helped me push Roland up the steep path to the church, which I wouldn't have managed otherwise. Pat spent quite a long time talking to various attenders. Roland got out of his chair and lay on the grass – while Tilly massaged his painful foot – watched somewhat enviously by some of the others.

8: Changes are on the Way

Early in September 2013, Pat and I were interviewed at Trevillis House, Liskeard by two psychiatrists and a cognitive therapist called Debbie. The upshot was that no evidence of stroke, tumour or other destructive or threatening abnormalities were found in Pat's CT scan, but the diagnosis was "mild cognitive impairment" associated with age and possible hypoxia due to a side effect of the general anaesthetic used when Pat's fractured wrist was repaired. This did not amount to a diagnosis of dementia but was nevertheless a degree of impairment exceeding what was normal for a person of Pat's age. We were advised that when the written diagnosis came through Pat would be obliged to notify DVLA and her motor insurance company. Their reactions would determine whether it was still legal and affordable for her to drive. As to the way forward, Pat was offered a place on an eight-week cognitive therapy course starting also at Trevillis House. She decided to attend the first session and see how it went.

Later that month I took Roland to his annual well-man clinic. His BP remained normal, and his weight had reduced by 2Kg since the previous year. His thyroid test result was also normal. I mentioned Roland's recently increased tendency to wee himself en route to the toilet. A quick urine test revealed proteins and leucocytes, so a sample was sent off to the lab to check for a urinary tract infection.

Our new case co-ordinator, Ernie, visited from Adult Social Care to update Roland's care plan and risk-assessment. From our point of view not much had changed since Lesley's previous in-depth review and the assistance with Roland's personal budget application. Recent news media implied that the Council was looking for ways to save money – particularly on transport. We took the opportunity to ask for one weekend per month for

Roland at Tregarne respite hostel rather than one weekend every two months.

Afterwards, Ernie rang to say Roland's personal budget would continue unchanged for 2014. I thanked him for his efforts. Pat and I attended a review meeting at MTL. Ernie said he would try to preserve Roland's entitlement to minibus transport but warned we might have to pay something towards this. Tilly was noted as Roland's emergency carer with no objection from Pat. Pat also made no objection to me mentioning her cognitive impairment – in the context of us applying for more respite care. Ernie said it might be helpful to have a carer's assessment.

I took Roland to the NHS dentist in February. Irma gave Roland a scale and polish as usual and found no problems – saying that he still had two milk-teeth firmly in place, but then she announced she was leaving the practice, which was disappointing.

Ernie and trainee Jill visited us at home regarding Roland's support plan and Pat's carer's assessment. The necessary paperwork was completed with significant assistance from Ernie.

In April Ernie rang and said we would have to pay £22 per week towards Gentian Centre transport – which might be billed separately. He also said that Roland's personal budget would be reduced somewhat to reflect reduced gym sessions. I reminded him that Roland would need transport back from Tregarne respite hostel in May and July.

Towards the end of the month, Tamsin and another woman visited us at home and quizzed us about Roland's finances. I explained that he received income support and DLA (Disability Living Allowance) but had no other income or property. They were not clear about how this information would affect the support provided by Cornwall Council – including Roland's personal budget – saying that £131 per week was considered the amount that a single man of Roland's age needed to live on.

At the beginning of May, Roland returned from MTL with a painful right ankle having fallen during the drama session. He said he had been running when he tripped. I cancelled the Gentian Centre that week as Roland was unable to walk. During the day he got through a lot of socks, trousers and T-shirts due to involuntarily peeing them while crawling towards a bucket we'd placed in the hall for this purpose. We unearthed the portable loo from the camping cupboard as it was much easier to sit on than a plasterer's bucket.

A week later Roland's ankle was still painful, so for Tamar Friends I wheeled him into the church hall in his chair. I tried taking him back to The Gentian Centre by mid-month, but he returned limping heavily again. There had apparently been no new mishap, but I decided that he would attend day centres with his wheelchair for the rest of the week. He was also due to play the lion in MTL's production of the Wizard of Oz, and he did this in his wheelchair wearing a lion hat and furry gloves with claws – pushed by a girl sporting a lion's tail. This was a rather complex production by Sue's MTL standards, and the audience of parents and carers was amusedly tolerant of the many hiccups, giving enthusiastic applause throughout. Sue came over to speak to us at the end of the show saying how pleased she was Roland had turned up despite his injury. I took the opportunity to emphasize how prone he was to falls.

When I collected Roland from The Gentian Centre on Friday of that week, Kit assured me that they had not encouraged Roland to walk on the previous Tuesday when he came home with renewed ankle pain – indeed they had used the Centre's wheelchair for a trip to Lux Park. As at MTL, I took the opportunity to emphasize once again how prone he was to injury from falls. Kit added that immediately prior to his recent fall at MTL Roland had been wearing floppy slippers that were intended to resemble lion paws. At the weekend I wheeled Roland to a travelling fair at Warfelton Field.

After watching for a while Roland braved the Twizzler and the Ghost Train and returned home happy.

At Tamar Friends, Roland won a Tamar Got Talent cup for his Ollie Murrs karaoke.

In mid-June, Roland returned from MTL rather subdued. We then noticed there was blood in his urine. I mentioned this to Tilly, and she urged me to take Roland to an emergency doctor without delay. The out of hours operator took me through a questionnaire then made Roland an appointment at Liskeard hospital at 9.50pm. We whizzed there by car and were seen almost immediately by a male doctor who was pleased to see we had come prepared with a urine sample in a sterile container. He dipped a diagnostic stick into the reddened urine then read off the result on a colour chart. This was positive for a UTI – possibly in the kidneys – so he immediately issued a 7-day course of Co-Amoxiclav - a strong antibiotic. We thanked him and returned home.

I cancelled The Gentian Centre. Roland stayed indoors resting – which was for the best as he needed to use his porta-loo frequently and had reduced appetite. Outside the weather was gloriously sunny with the temperature peaking at 25C. The following day Roland was slightly better – enough to spend time on his PS3 for a while – but he showed no inclination to go out despite the weather being brilliant.

In July I took Roland, Pat and Tilly to the Quest Festival. Tilly came with us to provide additional support. We all took part in Heiki's drumming circle – which was quite enjoyable – but no other workshops really took our fancy. Quest was fairly expensive for the four of us to attend that year – probably £100-plus with drinks from the bar and extra snacks. But Roland enjoyed it. When I was at the car with Roland, with the wheelchair and baggage ready to load. Pat had wandered off. I sent Tilly to find her – which she did – but Pat felt she had been left behind and was annoyed. Tilly gently defended my actions, and Pat settled down till the end of the journey – which was fast and trouble-free. It had been a rather odd Quest day – a "curate's egg" of a day, with some parts good and others not so good, but Roland was happy, which was the main thing.

Roland's 38th birthday came. He had a nice selection of cards, a new PS3 handset from Warren and some CDs from us. At teatime, we picked Tilly up from Landrake and set off for Jon and Mary's wedding party at Budleigh Farm near Bovey Tracey. Tables had been set up under cover of a long shed that was open on one side, and there was plenty of food and drink available – plus a hog being roasted over a giant gas barbecue. Eating, drinking and merrymaking continued till about 9pm when we gathered to play some drum rhythms – to generous applause from the non-drummers. Everyone sang happy birthday to Roland.

The gathering probably numbered about seventy people – with all ages and stages represented. After the drumming, an elderly guy blew a few tunes on a trumpet, followed by Mary's younger son playing the electric guitar. Around 10pm we walked to another field where there was an impressive display of fireworks. Roland and an old gent got a lift there and back in Adam's Landcruiser Amazon. It was oddly pleasant to hear its familiar diesel rattle – reminiscent of our smaller Toyota 4x4 - though as an old-style Amazon, it had the more powerful straight-six engine.

In mid-August, Ernie rang to say that the day-care rate we were paying to The Gentian Centre reflected the reduction in Roland's entitlement following the financial assessment a few months previously. He also said that Roland's respite had been re-instated to two nights per month. But when I rang Tregarne they not only hadn't been notified but also said that we were most unlikely to get a weekend allocation and that we would also be responsible for transport. However, in September, Ernie and a woman from Cornwall Council separately confirmed that taxis would be laid on to transport Roland to and from Tregarne.

I purchased a new extra-wide, heavy duty – but light alloy - wheelchair for Roland from CareCo – at a cost of £223 VAT-free in recognition of Roland's disabled status. It assembled easily and Roland admired it on his return from MTL.

On the 16th of September, Roland awoke pale and lethargic but insisted on going to the Gentian Centre, but we had to drive to Liskeard and pick him up mid-morning as they said he was unwell. The next day Roland was suffering from fatigue, diarrhoea and loss of appetite. He slept most of the day. I cancelled his day-centres and clubs for a few days. Carla from Tamar Friends said she knew of a few other people with Roland's symptoms. Two days later he was showing signs of recovery in terms of appetite but still spending the day on the settee.

By the 22nd he seemed a little better and his well-man clinic went okay. His blood pressure was 125/80 and his weight was down 2Kg on the previous year. Height was recorded at 5ft 2ins. Afterwards I contacted the NHS dentist and made a check-up appointment for him, but the following day his symptoms returned, and he was evidently out of sorts again – refusing breakfast – so I had to cancel his Gentian Centre session. He slowly perked up during the day, eating some leftover pizza for lunch and sausage and chips for his tea. Three days later, Roland was more or less back to normal, but he didn't want to go to The Gentian Centre. Kit didn't seem disappointed at this, so we made no objection to Roland staying at home for what now amounted to two week's absence from his day centres. At his request, we also cancelled his gym session on the following day. Nevertheless, Roland did choose to attend the out-and-about group's disco at Saltash Football Club – which he enjoyed despite having aching feet when he returned home.

Following a discussion with Warren about wills and trusts I emailed him a scanned version of the National Trustees for the Mentally Handicapped trust deed regarding Roland, to give him an idea of what was involved in leaving money to a person who lacked financial capacity.

Early in October, I took Roland to see the new dentist in the small surgery adjacent to the Saltash Medical Centre. The dentist set about a thorough examination of Roland's mouth – identifying a potential problem of loosening lower front teeth due to the formation of calculus at the gum line. She booked Roland in for another scale and clean in three months' time. It made me wonder how long the problem had been developing.

I phoned case co-ordinator Ernie to tell him Roland was being changed over to Employment Support Allowance (ESA/JSA) as a replacement for Income Support. The DWP said Roland would be getting an extra £20 per week – to be reviewed after three years.

At the end of October, I took Roland to see the practice nurse regarding the emergence of symptoms suggesting another UTI. The urine sample was inconclusive regarding an infection, but Roland was running a slight temperature (37.4c) so Trimethoprim was prescribed for a week. Back home, Roland demolished a good helping of liver, bacon and onions but later peed his bed in his sleep for the second night running. The medication cured the suspected infection after a few more days.

At the beginning of November, I took Roland and Pat drumming. Pat hadn't been to the Wednesday evening sessions for years, but she seemed to enjoy it. The class leader and others welcomed her back.

I took Roland to gym after several weeks' break. He returned tired but with a feeling of achievement. Ollie said his wealthy Jamaican uncle had died. He also mentioned that Derriford was currently snowed under with sufferers from chest problems – coughs and infections – which put my own persistent wheezy cough into some kind of context. Roland had a "flu-jab, which he bore well and returned home pleased with himself for being "brave".

Shortly before Christmas 2014, my mum Polly passed away at the age of 94. She had been fairly happy at the residential home and continued to enjoy being taken out on trips to the seaside by me and Tilly. The bond between her and Tilly grew stronger, and Tilly would visit in the evenings and help Polly with her personal hygiene routines and settle her for bed. Polly was very grateful for this loving attention as the care home staff tended to adopt a rather "one size fits all" impersonal approach. But Polly was becoming frailer and would sometimes fall after getting up from her chair, which led to her breaking a hip joint. She recovered surprisingly well from the repair operation, but it was a major shock to her system and Tilly sensed that Polly hadn't much longer to live.

One evening, Tilly "saw" Polly's mother and two gentlemen standing at the foot of Polly's bed. She mentally asked who they were, and they replied "Frank" and "George". Tilly said she was touched when the two men – appearing to her as solid, down to earth Yorkshiremen - thanked her for befriending Polly. Initially the men's names meant nothing to me, but when I looked, I found them in the family tree. They were Polly's uncles on her mother's side. Many years previously, Polly had said that in the 1920s some of her family had been into spiritualism, and it seemed that they were watching over her.

In the spring of 2014 Polly broke her other hip. She survived a second hip repair operation but needed nursing care thereafter. She was moved to a nearby nursing home only a few yards away from our home address. By this time, her vascular dementia was advanced and her short-term memory seriously impaired – but she still recognized family members and could carry on a conversation about everyday topics. Because the nursing home staff were overstretched, Polly would frequently be left alone in her room for hours at a time. We organized a rota so that Tilly, I and part-time private carers could keep her company. Increasingly it seemed that Polly was already in touch with the next world, although in her younger days she had always affected scepticism about such things. On one occasion I asked if she got lonely when there were no visitors. "Oh no" she said. "Plenty of people come to see me. The trouble is most of them are dead and when you ask them to fetch your cup of tea from across the room, they can't do it!"

On 13th December Polly was admitted to hospital with pneumonia. The male charge nurse said they would try intravenous antibiotics, but he made it clear there was a real risk Polly might not survive the infection. It seemed unclear whether it was helpful to stay so Tilly and I decided to leave. I kissed Polly's forehead, tried to reassure her before we left around midnight. Shortly after 2am I was woken from a deep sleep by a phone call from Derriford Hospital. A nurse broke the news that Polly had died peacefully at 1.49hrs. I texted Tilly and she quickly replied saying she already knew – Polly had "visited" her in Landrake and said goodbye.

9: Health Crises 2015 - 2017

With Polly's passing the last of our parents had gone, but life went on.

Tilly spoke to me earnestly about addressing the problem of Roland's obesity. He weighed 19 stone which I agreed was dangerous. Knowing that Pat would fiercely oppose imposition of a reduced intake, I decided to try and get the medical authorities involved in making appropriate changes to his diet – by way of "doctor's orders".

I made an appointment with our GP for Roland to see a dietitian and I left a message with Adult Social Care asking if Roland could swap his funded gym sessions for an extra day centre session.

Then I took Roland to see Robina at the health centre for a dietary health assessment. She agreed that, counting from 2011 when he weighed in at 19 ½ stone, Roland had been losing weight at a very modest 1 to 2Kg per year but had now reverted to his 2011 size and had his highest BMI to date. She read through a lifestyle note and detailed list of food intake I had prepared and made the following recommendations:

No biscuits or cakes to be included with dessert. Stop the daily apple juice and Nutri-grain bars. Cut potatoes down to three per meal. Home lunches should not include hot dogs – only microwaveable pizzas. Replace "full English" Sunday breakfast with cereal or a low-calorie substitute such as grilled mushrooms and tomatoes. Drink more water (zero-calorie flavoured water was okay). Whole bananas all right for desserts. Porridge okay for breakfast including a teaspoon of jam. Low-fat sandwiches fine for day centre lunches. Drink water before meals. Chew food thoroughly. Robina offered to contact Nola – a health trainer who might be able to recommend exercise routines in the absence of gym sessions.

I was beginning to feel the strain of looking after Roland and Pat and doing all the household chores, plus keeping up with my treasurer duties for a national charity and three local organizations. I wrote to all the chairpersons concerned explaining in detail my responsibilities regarding Roland's care and management of Pat's cognitive problems. All replied making helpful and sympathetic comments, but they didn't want me to step down.

Realizing that I had too many balls to juggle, Tilly offered a "meals on wheels" service, not just intended to change and support Roland's diet but to improve Pat's and mine too, given that use of convenience foods and takeaways was increasing so that I could cope.

Cornwall Council health advisor Nola made a home visit. We explained Roland's health background and she asked a series of lifestyle questions. In summary her suggestion was that Roland should try supervised aquarobics sessions. She said she would check the possibility of Monday morning sessions and get back to us.

In May, Ernie visited to update Roland's care plan. He worked from the previous version to save time. The significant changes stemmed from Pat's increasing frailty and consequently the shift of caring effort for Roland onto me. Pat agreed that this was the case – adding that, though she regretted it - she felt it was too risky for her to drive nowadays. Ernie offered to carry out a carer's assessment for me, and I accepted the offer. He said he would contact Nola and talk to her about the proposed arrangements for Roland's swimming sessions.

We all went to the Leisure Centre for Roland's first supervised aqua session with Nola. Pat watched from the café as I joined Nola and Roland in the pool. Nola took Roland through a number of simple exercises – finishing with him swimming four lengths in his leisurely style. Nola seemed impressed with Roland's abilities and confirmed she was happy to continue with the sessions – though there would be a gap of two weeks due to prior commitments. This suited us too.

I returned a call from Ernie about finalising the update to Roland's support plan and personal budget review – plus new carers' needs assessments for Pat and myself – as I was now recognised as a joint carer for Roland. An appointment was made for 15th June.

Pat was a little disconcerted when I broached the idea of Warren keeping her company for part of the time I would be at the weekend Astrological Association conference. I attempted to reassure her that she would not be expected to play hostess or look after Warren's children. As if on cue Warren rang in the evening and talked to me for over an hour about his concerns around Pat and the family. He ended by encouraging me not only to enlist his help with practical matters if the need arose but also to use him as an emotional sounding board if I became stressed by family problems. I thanked him for offering this support. Mindful that Tilly was thinking of emailing Warren with her assessment of the situation, I also took the opportunity to remind him that she was also the registered local emergency contact and was willing to look after Roland in the short term if Pat and I were unable to care for him for any reason.

Tilly wrote Warren an email, giving her take on our domestic issues:

Dear Warren,

Sharing another day with you all was memorable in many ways. I enjoyed getting to know you all a bit better as a result. I am glad too that you were able to talk to your dad about some very difficult concerns that will affect you all very deeply in the times ahead. As a family friend and observer, always willing to offer unconditional help, I trust it does not feel presumptuous to voice some thoughts that keep crossing my mind and heart. I feel sure that our concerns are similar.

Conscious of the ever-increasing support needs at home, which your dad is trying to adjust to, has motivated me to raise the subject with you. The support for your mum lies with Robert and you, hopefully in times ahead aided by outside professional care staff, as I feel it is not my place to be at your dad's side in that way. Whatever relationship your parents can enjoy now, it is still an intimate one shaped by a longstanding partnership with special bonds. Nevertheless, I am still concerned for you all and may be able to lighten the load in other ways. Your Mum does enjoy the ambience of my Landrake home and the attention of the cats!

The following weighs heavily on my mind and fills me with sadness for you all: I trust my words will not upset you, not my intention:

I sense your mum feeling very frightened, worried and insecure about the increasing loss of her mental and physical faculties. She knows she is diminishing slowly but surely from the person you know her to be and the roles she played in all your lives. Sad for grandchildren Charlie and Mitzi too who will not experience her vitality and love for long. How much you involve them in the changes ahead will be a difficult decision to make for you. I imagine Charlie will be asking questions, as he is beginning to relate well to your Mum. Any hands-on help that you offer, whether it involves your family or not will nevertheless impact on you all.

I believe your dad to be physically strong with enough love and patience (the latter he says our friendship has improved) to try and cope with the care responsibilities for both Pat and Roland. However, the ever-increasing isolation and lack of intellectual stimulation will affect him mentally and emotionally. He is already beginning to feel the reduction in his personal time and space to deal with anything outside the home, given your dad is hardly able to go anywhere or do anything without your mum being part of it somehow; or if he does it causes upsets. Given the offices he holds and the admin work that he needs to do (your company's accounting included which he enjoys), it will prove increasingly difficult to find the time and space for juggling it all, causing pressure and frustration. So, he does need your support to give him time out to attend social/business meetings and conferences. I have a feeling your support for the AA conference could pave the way for your mum to accept carers eventually coming into the home in the future to support her and your dad.

And then there is Roland, already aware and puzzled. How will he cope with what is to come? Your dad is reluctant to involve *support agencies for your mum, although there has been a lot of research into this area of mental health and support is available. I can understand his concern about potentially having things taken out of his hands. Roland's care is already monitored; worst case scenario means at some point the joint care needs of two vulnerable people will prove too much. Social Services will then intervene where Roland is concerned, which is not in his best interest or your parents. However as long as I am fit and healthy, Roland will not go into care by default. I take my emergency carer's responsibilities for him very seriously and thankfully we have a bond already. Therefore, having the skills and energy, I would be willing to take on the care of Roland if it was a help, and Robert would accept in order to continue to care for Pat. He knows from our shared Polly experience that my offer when it comes to it would be genuine and sincere, which means I will see that through whatever it entails with no strings attached. During my career as a teacher and community worker I have taught and supported people such as Roland on programmes that improved their living skills, thus increasing their independence, so not a daunting task for me.*

Well, time will give us the answers to all our concerns. I am sure both you and Robert will find the love expressed in positive and constructive handling of whatever evolves. Life is precious, reminding us about what is important to do now and what is not. My support will always be there too should you need it, I leave that to you.

Love to all. Tilly

I took Roland for his annual thyroid sample. He was nervous because of the needle but coped well. The result was "normal".

His next swim session with Nola followed a developing pattern of more lengths swum each time, and time in the water of nearly one hour. Once back home it was clear Roland was tired by his efforts, and after lunch he had a long snooze.

Weighed Roland – just over 18 stone. Tilly rang and kindly invited Roland, Pat and me to a meal on his 39th birthday. She was very pleased to hear of his continued healthy weight loss but thought his diet could be improved further. Tilly noted that

Roland had an aversion to fresh vegetables and opined his intake of sugar and starchy foods, along with fast food, was still too high. She had studied and taught nutrition in her younger days and came up with a way forward. The approach was basically to include freshly cooked vegetables in sauces. This worked because Roland loved sauces and gravies. Tilly started to cook our main meals using only fresh ingredients including vegetable-enriched gravies and she delivered them to the house in "cauldrons" containing a variety of foods for all of us for a week. One portion would be eaten on the day and the others went into the freezer.

Initially, Pat was dubious. She regarded provision of food as her province and queried Tilly's involvement. Pat had already but rather reluctantly accepted Tilly's support of Roland as she could see that he liked her. Another major concession was giving Tilly a key to the house in her role as emergency carer. No other non-residents, apart from Warren, had a key. So, handing over responsibility for preparing main meals as well was a big deal. Slowly however, with a few disputes along the way, Pat came to accept this additional help. The food was good, and we all enjoyed eating it. The deliveries of cauldrons became an established routine.

Came Roland's birthday and we all set off for Tilly's where she regaled us with a sumptuous roast beef lunch and all the trimmings. She had also filled some balloons with helium, and we released these – whereupon they flew off in a westerly direction. One balloon, on which I had written "Mooneroids for ever" (in reference to Roland, Tilly and me because we shared a particular configuration of planets in our star charts), got stuck in a tall tree. Eventually it freed itself and followed its companions. Tilly remarked that this was quite telling – adding that the Cosmos had a sense of humour. After this we played Scrabble in the chapel yard.

It was very pleasant in the sunshine and gentle breezes, and we continued until nearly five in the afternoon. Tilly presented Roland with a healthy carrot cake and some simple presents – and Pat received a big bunch of flowers.

Following another consultation with Adult Social Care, a revised care plan was put into place making me Roland's primary carer. It then became startlingly evident that this shift of

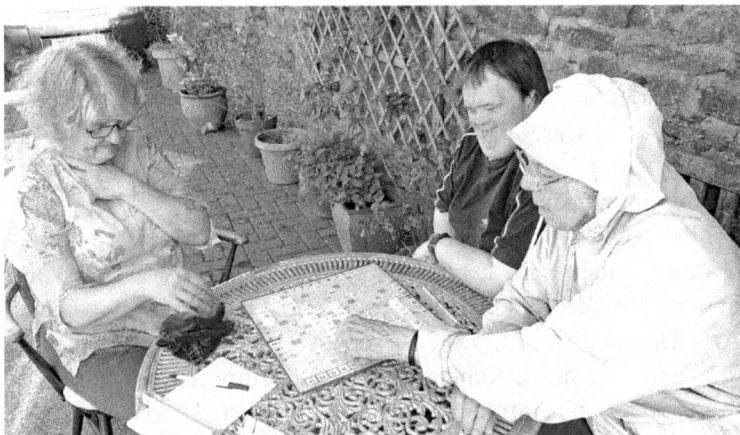

TILLY, ROLAND AND PAT PLAYING SCRABBLE: 2015

responsibility had occurred none too soon, as Pat was briefly hospitalised while I was away at the 2015 AA conference; she had turned up at the local health centre in a confused state while Warren was travelling down from Somerset to look after her. I returned from the conference post haste and conferred with the hospital medics. Pat was diagnosed with small vessel disease (SVD) of the brain. Warren stayed for a couple of days to give additional support.

I began to feel overstressed due to lack of sleep and worry about Pat's worsening mental health.

At the beginning of December, I arranged to meet with Tilly to discuss how best to organize care arrangements for the future. Carer Carrie arrived promptly to sit with Pat and Roland for the evening and I left them setting up the table to do jigsaws.

It was pleasant sitting talking to Tilly but as we sat overlooking the river Tamar and the lights of Saltash beyond, I began to feel oddly sad. Tilly sensed this and gently quizzed me about how I was feeling. I found it hard to put into words. The nearest I could get was a sense of regret at leaving the world – as if someone close was dying. I said that the feeling reminded me of a dream my brother John had after our dad's death. To the accompaniment of classical music, Gil had visualised the world dropping away beneath him, with its lights obscured by mists and gradually growing fainter until they were gone. With hindsight I feel this was a premonition.

Later that month Pat was diagnosed with Alzheimer's disease. Adult Social Care confirmed we were entitled to 36 nights per annum respite from Roland's care though there was a potential impact on his benefits.

Pat could still enjoy outings, so we went to see Roland in a drama production of Cinderella at Morley Tamblyn Lodge, also in a medley of I'm a Celebrity and Jungle Book at the St Austell Arts Theatre.

Dementia nurse Rene arrived for a follow-up session to the diagnostic appointment with psychiatrist Dr Lombard in November 2015. She started by asking Pat if she wanted to try medication that might improve her cognitive skills – particularly memory. After we asked about its success rate, side-effects and limitations and discovered that it could not cure or retard the progress of Alzheimer's. Pat decided she would embark on a three-month trial during which her reactions to the drugs would be monitored and if considered appropriate, the dose could be ramped up. This was conditional on her heart being healthy, and I agreed to make an appointment for an ECG to be carried out locally. Also mentioned were memory cafes, "AGE(UK)", "Living Well" and other bodies organizing activities aimed at mitigating the socially isolating effects of the disease on sufferers.

The discussion then turned to the impact of Pat's condition on her and the family. Rene approved the involvement of a limited number of ad hoc private sitters, saying that as the disease progressed, familiarization with the experience of accepting a small number of regular sitters was a stress-reducing preliminary to the likely need for longer periods of family respite later on. Not only were NHS home-support services very stretched but also NHS sitters tended to have a formulaic approach to their duties and there was no guarantee that the same sitters would be allocated from session to session – thus losing the advantages of familiarity.

Clearly uncomfortable with my absences, Pat remarked that I was constantly going out for long periods of time. Rene answered for me, saying that it was understandable that Pat should regard me as "her everything" – but that I needed time out to maintain mental stimulation and health by pursuing my interests. Rene added that clock-watching would inevitably make the sittings drag for Pat and it would be preferable for her to find activities that required some attention and concentration – such as light conversation and jigsaws etc. I explained that we were already working on this.

I asked Rene if, given the dependence of our little household on my continuing health and well-being, there was a way conceptually to join up local authority learning disability and geriatric care services in our case. She made a note of Roland's case co-ordinator's details - and said she would contact him. She also said she would make a referral to the Cornwall Carer's service on my behalf.

After Rene left, I took Pat to lunch at Seaton beach. It remained windless and sunny throughout, and we were able to sit outside and enjoy basking in the rays for half an hour. Unexpectedly, the Gentian Centre crew turned up with Roland. He wanted to stay with his group for lunch, so we said our hellos and left them to it.

Early in 2016 I took Roland and Pat to the Theatre Royal in Plymouth to see Cinderella – with discounted tickets courtesy of the Out and About group. After a minor hassle persuading staff that we had a wheelchair space reserved we settled down to watch the show. For a while the amplified sound and flashing lights unsettled Pat but eventually, she began to enjoy the performance – with Gok Kwan as a creditable fairy godmother and a ventriloquist Buttons. Pat had a very vocal wobble at the end when fumbling for her bag and coat prior to leaving the crowded auditorium – but calmed down on the way home. This episode reminded me of a remark Tilly had made that it would become more and more difficult for me to manage both Roland and Pat on outings as time went on.

A few days later, news came that Pat's older brother Seb had died at his home in Yorkshire. Pat did not seem to understand this, and she declined an invitation from her nephew Simon to attend Seb's funeral.

Pat experienced hallucinatory side effects from the anti-psychotic medication, so I discontinued it with medical agreement.

We continued going on family trips. For an outing to Paignton Zoo, I loaded two wheelchairs into the car, and together with Roland and Pat, and Tilly as support for Roland, we set off to rendezvous with the Out and About group. We arrived with time to spare. Once Una had paid for us to go in, Tilly and I took turns to push Roland and Pat around the zoo in the wheelchairs. Both got out when gradients were steep. This arrangement worked well as it tided Pat over the morning period when she tended to be more confused and lacking in energy. In fact, as the afternoon progressed, she was bubbling over with enthusiasm in a rather nonsensical way and didn't want to go home.

On a sunny May morning I drove Pat and Roland to Landrake where we collected Seb en-route as additional support for Pat, then joined the Out and About group at Cotehele Quay for the start of a canoeing trip. We arrived around noon to find several members already gathering near the canoes. There was time to grab a quick sandwich lunch before it was time to don our buoyancy aids and take our places in the boats. Most of the big Canadian-style canoes were rafted together in pairs for stability but there were a few singles. Pat, Seb and another woman had a single while I, Roland, plus four others occupied one of the doubles. There were probably around forty people in the party – with three supervisors from Tamar Trails. Around 1.30pm we set off for Calstock. There was an amusing level of inefficiency in the paddling and steering – but speed was not of the essence – so we were happy to reach the Calstock viaduct about ninety minutes into the trip. Having gathered round the next bend in the river, we returned to Calstock and joined the landlubbers ashore. There we enjoyed light refreshments in the sunshine for about half an hour before clambering back into our boats. We reached our home port of Cotehele around 4.30pm. Having been quiet if rather fidgety throughout the trip, Pat had a minor wobble when ashore about the money in her handbag, but she soon calmed down again. Though standing on the flat ground of the quay, Pat suddenly lost her balance at one point – and would have fallen if Seb hadn't caught her arm and steadied her. She'd done no paddling because of a tender right wrist so was unlikely to have been tired due to any exertion. Roland needed a partial change of clothing, so we were soon back at Landrake where Tilly treated us to tea and lemon drizzle cake. It had been a brilliant day out.

Roland was granted exemption from jury service following a summons to take part!

Community psychiatric nurse Brenda made a home visit. She and colleague Molly gently questioned Pat and me about how we were coping. I tried to communicate my sense of vulnerability being the sole carer for Pat and Roland, my concern about the impending loss of Seb as Pat's "star carer", Pat's unwillingness to engage with care providers in general, and the difficulty in dealing with the inevitable but erratic development of her Alzheimer's. Pat remained calm throughout and did her best to answer questions. There was no discussion of residential care options – but quite a lot about local day-care organizations. Brenda also said she would consult Dr Lombard about prescribing Metazepine – which combined sedative and anti-depressant properties.

Over the next couple of weeks, I looked into residential care options for Pat. I phoned Tamar House, Saltash and St Winolls in Polbathic, and they both said it would be all right for us to visit. Celia from Coombe House at Liskeard returned my call. She took Pat's details and said that three recent deaths had created a vacancy at the home. I emailed Warren, Seb and Tilly suggesting that Seb and I take Pat to see Coombe House.

I mentioned my brief research into Dementia Care Matters and Butterfly Homes to Tilly. Warren replied to my email agreeing Coombe House was worth a second look and that I should include Pat and Seb.

There followed disturbed nights due to Pat wandering in and out of the bedroom talking to herself and rattling items on the bedside tables. She kept seeking reassurances of love and support - wobbling between saying that caring for her and Roland was becoming too much for me, fearfulness about being "cast off", and jealousy of my attachments to other people and activities.

She started obsessing about her handbag and its contents, saying that I or persons unknown had removed money and other items. After physically going through the contents with her a couple of times I disengaged from the debate.

Leading up to the evening meal Pat was in an accusing mood, saying that I was denying her use of her money and other possessions. This briefly morphed into a kind of sarcasm, such as when I reminded her that her meal was on a tray and she should eat it before it got cold, she responded by asking if I was sure that it was hers and would I really allow her to eat it.

She returned to the subject of her handbag and purse, and their contents. For around half an hour she was convinced there were cats or other animals in her bag which needed to be rescued, repeatedly asking me to go with her to the local police station or church to hand them over for safekeeping. I repeated that I couldn't see any cats or other animals and the bizarre idea slowly subsided.

The upshot of conversations with Tilly was that she thought I needed to make up my own mind about the suitability or otherwise of care homes and decide for myself when to take Pat on visits, as she thought the latter were likely to be problematic at best. This was fair enough.

Seb agreed to doing day and night shifts with Pat at home for a while, and Roland and I stayed with Tilly at her home in Landrake. This allowed me to catch up with some much-needed sleep as I was providing most of the transport to and from Roland's day centres and had nearly dozed off at the wheel a few times. Warren offered to visit Coombe House with me and Pat in mid-January. In the interim, Tilly and I visited two care homes – in rural Cornwall and in Plymouth. Neither seemed ideal.

I received a copy of a letter from CPN Brenda to Dr Maddie relating her findings from meeting Pat and me. The content reflected my initial letter to Dr Maddie, adding that different medications for Pat were being considered and that arrangements might be made regarding daytime respite for me.

At the end of our stay with Tilly the MTL taxi returned Roland to Landrake, and I took him home. Pat was initially bewildered by my return and appeared to confuse me with Seb. At one point she asked me if I was the man who was "married to himself" which I thought was oddly witty – if unintentionally so.

At bedtime, Pat started talking about there being another woman in the house whom she regarded as a threat. Pat mentioned a boy who accompanied the woman and was also "dangerous". Pat was concerned for her safety and for Roland's – and asked me for reassurance that I wouldn't let the woman kill her. I replied by saying that Roland was proof against such things, but I would protect them both anyway. In reply to me saying that I hadn't seen another woman in the house Pat said a couple of times that I didn't seem to believe her, but the threat was real. I accompanied Pat around the house as she peered carefully into each room – but she didn't see the woman or boy. I wondered whether the mysterious woman and boy were distorted perceptions of Tilly and Seb but mention of Tilly's name produced no response. I asked Pat what the woman looked like. She thought for a moment then said the woman wore a uniform – like a nurse's – and was carrying a hypodermic needle. We had recently watched an episode of Doc Martin – but there were no threatening female characters or boys in the storyline.

Early in February there was a home visit from psychiatrist Dr Freda. She introduced herself, then gently questioned Pat to test her level of understanding of a number of issues related to her daily life. She then turned to me and embarked on much more detailed enquiries about Pat's recent medical history and symptoms. Seb chipped in occasionally with helpful anecdotal information. Dr Freda complimented us on our approach to caring for Pat. She then talked about possible medication options. Drugs discussed were Pregabalin, Memantine, Metazepine and Lorazepam. Before any of these could be prescribed, blood tests would be required to establish base levels of organic function – followed by similar tests at monthly intervals. Dr Freda also recommended a "falls risk assessment" to be carried out at home and thought that a SALT assessment (re swallowing reflex) might be indicated in the medium term.

The initial conclusions were that, provided blood tests were satisfactory, Memantine would be tried to reduce emotional distress and hallucinations, and a supply of Lorazepam would be prescribed for use only in crisis situations as a fast-acting anxiolytic. Pat coped quite well with being questioned and being talked about and was fairly calm when the doctor departed. I was preparing to return to Landrake, while Dr Freda wrote giving an up-to-date assessment of Pat's condition and recommending medication to treat the Alzheimer's symptoms. I copied it to Warren, Seb and Tilly.

In March 2017, CPN Brenda visited to review Pat's situation and stayed for about an hour-and-a-half. She asked a lot of questions to ascertain if there were any changes since her last visit. She noted that Pat had begun taking Memantine and said it would take a while to kick in. I said her restlessness, confusion and anxiety had not gone away but Seb and I had been able to manage Pat's care without too many crises. I mentioned the plan for Roland to move to the bungalow in a few months' time and Brenda considered that the 'loss' of Roland and departure of Seb would need careful handling to avoid upsetting Pat. I agreed and said that efforts would be made to manage the transition with minimum disruption – adding that we were in the process of recruiting replacement carers.

At the end of May, Dr Freda arrived for another psychiatric appointment. She explained that her visit had been prompted by our GP referring to problems with the medication. Dr Freda asked Pat some very simple questions: the current date, her age, the number of her children, who I was and so on, hardly any of which Pat could answer correctly. She then asked me for my account of recent events. I explained my reasons for stopping Pat's medication (dizziness and unsteadiness at night) and the doctor accepted these. I added that Pat seemed to have become calmer and less anxious and restless, though I said it was likely I was sleeping through a lot of her night-wandering round the house – especially as approximately half the time she chose to sleep in a little room adjacent to the master bedroom that the carers called her "den". Commenting that she was surprised at how well I was coping, the psychiatrist went on to say that it was possible Pat's restlessness and anxiety would return and that I shouldn't hesitate to contact the psychiatric team if this happened. Dr Freda added that she would be taking up a post in Devon and that her post in

Cornwall would not be filled but CPN Brenda would still be on the team under Dr Lombard. She would suggest to Brenda that Pat be discharged from their caseload and would not receive further review visits unless I requested them. I said this was okay by me – adding that I had support from a small team of private carers which was allowing me valuable respite. The evening passed fairly quietly – in contrast to the aftermath of previous "official" visits when Pat would usually become anxious and agitated.

***

One sunny day, I took Pat and Roland for lunch at the Plymouth Barbican. I shared a bacon, cheese and pineapple baguette with Pat, and Roland had a chicken salad bap, all washed down with tea and coffee. After three hours, both Pat and Roland verged on becoming unmanageable due to various gripes - e.g., Pat needing a toothpick and saying her desire to stay all day should take precedence over Roland's wishes, and Roland having had enough of walking about and the hot sunshine. A kindly shop assistant gave Pat a kebab stick to pick her teeth with – and two other people made space for us at a Cap'n Jasper's table and bench – so we must have looked a needy bunch. Overall though, we enjoyed the outing.

Both Pat and Roland were a bit fractious leading up to the evening meal – possibly due to fatigue. I fought back mounting impatience while Pat fluttered around asking nonsensical questions just as I was trying to get things done. After the meal Roland occupied himself quite happily but Pat hovered, inventing reasons why I should stop what I was trying to do – and dance attendance on her. As bedtime approached, Pat asked a few times if she was going to die during the night, then asked for a drink of water then asked me if it was poisoned. She settled down around midnight.

By mid-July, carer Annie said she was coming to the view that there had been an escalation in Pat's Alzheimer's. This was based on increased confusion at night e.g., making more nonsensical comments, forgetting where the toilet was and preparing to pee/defaecate in the kitchen in a bowl, with incontinence generally becoming more of an issue. Also reportedly trying to clean her teeth with a scrubbing brush. I fitted two grab-handles in the toilet in the hope of reducing Pat's risk of falls in that location. I tried to explain to a concerned Roland that his mum was ill and couldn't help her behaviour.

At the end of July, I took Pat to see Dr Sheila. The purpose of the appointment was to seek advice about ongoing treatment following the increased falls risk at home, and Pat's occasional episodes of incontinence. The discussion turned into a review of Pat's medical history including the progression of diagnoses since 2013 from mild cognitive impairment, via small vessel disease of the brain, to the Alzheimer's in 2015 and its development to date. I listed changes I had noticed over the last twelve months, such as increased confusion, unsteadiness, anxiety and fatigue, loss of appetite and weight, deterioration of eyesight, restlessness at night and drowsiness during the day.

Dr Sheila said she was willing to refer Pat for a "falls assessment" and "incontinence assessment". But in view of her age and the evident progression of her Alzheimer's, the doctor questioned the value of additional "pokings and proddings" – especially as, when compos mentis several years previously, Pat had declined cataract surgery due to anxiety about spending time in hospital. I added that I had first noticed mental impairment after Pat had undergone general anaesthesia – and was now very concerned about a further impact of anaesthetics on her impaired brain function.

The doctor asked me what I would want done if I or a carer were to find Pat sitting on the toilet unconscious and was unable to rouse her. This seemed an odd question to ask me out of the blue, but it eerily recalled the circumstances leading to Pat's mum's death – when she was found slumped in a chair and her husband couldn't wake her. It turned out that mum had suffered a severe stroke and she'd died in hospital a few weeks later.

It seemed highly unlikely that Dr Sheila would know about Pat's mum, so my initial response was to say that we would cross that bridge when we came to it. She retorted that it would not be a kindness to allow paramedics to make heroic efforts to revive Pat if there was no realistic prospect of recovery, yet this is what would happen unless there was documentation in place to allow a natural death.

Having witnessed her mum's lingering death in hospital, being unable to move, speak or swallow, I agreed that Pat would not want to share a similar fate. I added that Pat had given me and Warren an LPA in respect of health and welfare. Dr Sheila said she would sign a treatment escalation plan (TEP) form stating that her medical judgement was in favour of not resuscitating Pat if she suffered a cardio-respiratory collapse. The doctor issued the completed form to me with the instruction that it be displayed in a prominent position at home and that close relatives and carers should be made aware of its content and location and should draw it to the attention of paramedics/doctors in the event of a medical emergency. I attached the TEP form to the memory photo-board in the lounge – and a pdf of it to an email sent to Warren, and to sitters Annie, Iggie and Petra and I also copied it to Tilly.

I was left with the feeling that this had been a portentous day. I couldn't resist the logic of what Dr Sheila had said and done, but it somehow made the prospect of Pat's demise more of an inescapable reality and made it feel closer. I remembered a similar conversation with doctors in September 2012 about Polly when she was in the care home. The appropriate paperwork was completed but apparently not shown to paramedics by the staff when Polly suffered a cardiac arrest after fracturing her right hip in March 2014. They revived her only for her to continue, bedridden, for a further nine months until she finally died in a nursing home in December 2014 after a series of chest infections. I didn't want Pat to endure something similar.

Warren replied to my email re the Dr Sheila consultation:

"Yes, I can understand you feeling that such decisions / conversations are portentous. Emotional and sad as the topic is, I have to agree that facing the prospects of such decisions is a bravely positive step. I only remember the case of Polly that you spoke about, but in my making of things, I found the very sight of her lying in hospital seemingly trapped in a propped up, but ultimately broken body, much worse that the thought of her actually being dead (released). In similar circumstances I would prefer that my mum didn't suffer that end for the sake of preserving life at all costs - very sad thoughts, but worth facing just in case it one day helps."

On 2nd August it was Roland's 41st birthday. I weighed him – just under 13 stones. We went drumming in the evening. At close of play Roland did an amazing ten-minute solo on the big drums which everyone applauded. He and "Bodmin Dave" indulged in a whimsical episode of naming a list of fruits in comical voices – which left leader Jon somewhat nonplussed.

Well Done Roland!

Roland has been slowly loosing weight for a couple of years now and is very proud of himself and wants to tell everyone he has currently lost 6 stone and is still counting.

Roland slowly increased his exercise and overcame his fear of vegetables. He also has amazing will power and refuses sugary snacks, sweets and cakes.

The newsletter group have researched some fun facts about the 6 stone Roland has lost and it is the equivalent to a massive 68 basket balls!

MTL NEWSLETTER: JUNE 2017

Later that month Warren emailed saying he'd enjoyed a recent visit and remarked that Pat and I looked less stressed than on his previous visit. I thought it was time I emphasized how stressful I found coping with everyday life at home so explained:

"Yes, it was good to see you all and I thought the visit went well. Glad your mum and I didn't look too knackered! She was not trying to do too much – which is important – but we had a restless night after you left. At 4 am she got up and was walking round the house turning all the lights on and saying it was daytime and we all needed to be up. In vain I pointed to the clock and the darkness outside. In the calmest of voices, she kept saying that she knew it was daytime whatever I might say. This went on until Roland woke up and joined in my attempts to persuade her that she should go back to bed. It was an odd feeling talking to someone who was asserting black was white in the face of the facts. I tried turning the excess lights off and going back to bed but she simply came into the bedroom, turned the bright ceiling light back on, and told me it was most important I get up. She added that it was impossible to turn the lights off once she'd turned them on. At length I persuaded her to take a Zopiclone sleeping pill and she gradually became drowsy, eventually allowing herself to be persuaded into bed and falling asleep half an hour later."

I'm sure you can imagine that, although your Mum is displaying less confrontational behaviour at present, nowadays I can't relax when she is awake as she follows me wherever I go. Neither can I sleep soundly because I know she might get up at any time and get into difficulties of one type or another. So, although your family visit was a welcome distraction, I am in a state of tension at some level all the time. The reality is that my wife is no longer my partner and can never be so again. The emotional and practical support from Tilly during respite breaks is enabling me to keep going and get useful work done but even this doesn't allow me to achieve a regular sleep pattern because the breaks don't go on long enough. Roland's relocation to the bungalow is primarily aimed at developing his independent living skills. I agree it's very unlikely he will ever be truly independent, but the nearer he can comfortably approach this the better it will be for him when family and friends are no longer able to take an active role in caring for him. Some of his acquaintances have been in sheltered housing for years and they seem to be happy enough – so I have to hope that the same will apply to Roland. Certainly, Tilly and I are doing our best to make the bungalow a pleasant place to live in and, as you saw, it is beginning to look like a home now and will be a super little place when the renovation is completed. I'm also hoping, with Tilly looking after Roland, that a spin-off will be more time and energy for me to care for Pat. Relief from the necessity of getting up and functioning at 7am irrespective of what has happened during the night will be a real bonus. Likewise, being able to take Pat out at any time without the worry of leaving Roland "home alone" or needing to be back in time to meet his day-centre transport every weekday will be a great help. At the very least, the relief from being a double-carer should extend the period I'm able to continue supporting Pat at home. Of course, we won't know what emotional impact Roland's move will have on Pat until it happens. But I have noticed that her focus is increasingly on her own perceived needs so my feeling is that she will sometimes realize Roland is absent and miss him, whilst at other times not questioning his absence. We shall see. I am reasonably confident that Roland will adapt better, as his understanding of circumstances is now superior to his mum's – plus he gets on very well with Tilly and trusts her."

Tilly produced a useful timeline plan for Roland's move to the bungalow and the consequent changes to day centre transport arrangements. I emailed it to Ernie and to the Gentian Centre. I did the necessary admin to register Roland's change of address with the benefits agencies. This was always a time-consuming process as the agency staff usually wanted to speak to Roland for verification, but he struggled to answer their questions.

In September, prompted by a renewal invitation letter from the DVLA, Pat signed a form voluntarily surrendering her driving licence for medical reasons.

Pat had a fall in the kitchen. This caused a hairline crack in her pelvic ramus but there was no treatment available apart from painkillers and careful mobilization, and the fracture healed naturally.

Warren visited with his children Charlie and Mitzi towards the end of October. As teatime approached Tilly dropped Roland off outside and walked in. Pat seemed pleased to see him in a vague sort of way but didn't interact. Roland greeted his mum and looked round with a flicker of interest at the altered appearance of the lounge – but then settled on his favourite couch and watched the children play. Mitzi played with nurse and doctor figures and busied herself applying bandages to the adults, pretending to take their blood pressures and using the toy stethoscope, while Charlie played on his iPad. Later Warren, Roland and Charlie wrestled for control of toy hypodermics; each resisting being "jabbed". Warren and family stayed until 8pm then departed. It had been an enjoyable visit, and it was significant because Pat and Roland had been re-united temporarily without any apparent upset.

Afterwards I had a long telephone conversation with Tilly during which she related in detail a discussion she'd had with

Warren after his visit. She had taken the opportunity to address all the family issues she thought might be troubling him – and believed she had made progress.

Near the end of October, occupational therapist, Edward, from domiciliary support visited and fitted a seat on the bath so that showers could be taken in a sitting position. Additional handrails were fitted on the stairs and in the bathroom. A slightly raised toilet seat was provided to make it easier to stand up from.

In early November, Roland departed for The Gentian Centre and thence to a respite weekend at Tregarne, and Izzie arrived to look after Pat for the weekend because Tilly and I had to attend two days of meetings in London. However, we had to return early as Roland had fainted at Tregarne and was taken to hospital for observation. Seb, who had been on standby for Tilly at the bungalow during our time away, went to keep him company. The medics found nothing serious amiss and concluded that a combination of mild dehydration and a UTI had lowered blood pressure and caused the faint. Roland returned home with a prescription for antibiotics.

Roland had suffered five urinary tract infections in the period 2015 to 2017. These were all dealt with using prescription antibiotics. We assumed Roland was prone to these because of his underdeveloped Genito-urinary system – his very short and narrow urethra - which had the side-effect of making it difficult for him to fully empty his bladder.

Occupational therapist Edward rang asking how Pat and I were getting on and I said the handrails were useful. He asked about the use of Lorazepam as this could lead to unsteadiness. I explained I had used it only once – and Zopiclone only rarely.

After Edward left, I watched TV with Pat until 11pm. She said a few times that she missed a bespectacled man who slept in the double bedroom – as he was kind and helpful. She was definite that it wasn't me!

10: Care for the Carers

2017 - 2019

Pat and I celebrated our birthdays in mid-November 2017, but the day after mine I suffered an acute and prolonged episode of breathlessness. Fearing collapse, I rang Tilly at the bungalow and she drove me to hospital. Pat and Roland tagged along. After a battery of tests, it emerged that I had a form of pneumonia. Strong antibiotics were prescribed, and I was discharged with instructions to have complete rest for at least a week and advice that it would take several months for me fully to recover. An uncomprehending Pat was moved to a care home on a temporary basis to give me respite but she broke out during the first night and ended up in hospital where aggressively demented behaviour led to her being sectioned under the Mental Health Act. She was transferred to Garner psychiatric ward in Bodmin hospital where efforts were made to stabilize her with a cocktail of anti-psychotic and anxiolytic drugs. The process took seven months during which I was a regular visitor and Warren also visited when he could.

Looking back on the previous two years I was grateful that Roland had remained relatively healthy apart from the urinary tract infections, as Pat's increasing frailty had put an unsustainable strain on my own health despite the support that I received from Tilly, family members and paid helpers. Also, Roland's weight had gradually reduced from 19 stone to nearer ten stone as a result of eating the healthy diet devised by Tilly.

I considered the future of our family home. I reflected that my attitude to the house had shifted away from trying to renovate it - towards clearance and selling up with or without renovation.

At the bungalow, Tillie continued working on Roland's toilet training (a long-standing issue) and other basic living skills.

In a conversation with manager Tricia at Bodmin Hospital she commented that she didn't know how I'd lasted so long as I had as Pat's carer. She went on to say that, as a Section Three detainee, Pat might be eligible to have financial assistance with her care that was not means-tested under S.117 of the Mental Health Act. She gave me a leaflet explaining this and a printout of nursing homes in East Cornwall. Tricia said that an ordinary residential care home would not be suitable and that it would have to be a nursing home with a locked door policy.

In mid-January 2018 I attended an aftercare planning meeting at Bodmin. The first issue agreed was that Pat did not have capacity to participate in the after-care planning – so it became a "best interests" session. I answered questions about Pat's recent mental health history and made it clear that I could not resume caring for Pat at home – Brenda chipped in with the comment that it was the stress of caring that had led to my pneumonia. It was decided that S.117 funding would be provided to meet the cost of a dementia nursing home placement – and this non-means tested funding was reviewed annually. I decided to visit nursing homes of my choice and report back to the hospital with a shortlist while treatment for Pat continued in hospital.

After the meeting, I went to Garner Ward to see Pat. She was alert and talkative in a quirky way. She referred to the other patients as "jellifants", a talkative male as a "double-quack", and a woman she didn't like as a "cork-head". Pat kept wanting to move around and sit in different seats. She referred to me as her dad a few times and referred to her mother as "a bit crackers". Warren rang and I updated him with details of the Bodmin Hospital meeting.

I rang Case Co-ordinator, Ernie. He said Roland was due for a review, but Adult Social Care were currently short-staffed and likely to remain so, and thus only had time for emergency care situations. I briefly explained that Pat was no longer able to able to care for Roland in any capacity and that Tilly was his home carer. Ernie recommended that we keep a diary of Roland's needs and his developing self-help abilities. He also agreed to send us a list of residential homes and sheltered housing options for us to look at in advance of Roland's future move out of home care. Ernie added that if the family were able to contribute towards accommodation costs this afforded a wider choice. Adult Social Care would always provide accommodation in case of emergency i.e., if no relatives or friends were able to provide care.

The next morning Roland got up early and made himself a cheese and ham toastie using the new machine. I prepared the evening meal for Roland and me. As usual he helped lay the table plus drying up and putting the dishes away after I had washed up. He also did a couple of wash-loads and tumble-drying sessions unbidden. Roland showered and packed his bag ready for the Gentian Centre.

Exhausted by the pressures of supporting me as well as caring for Roland, Tilly developed a kidney infection that followed a number of urinary tract infections. She then developed shingles leading to acute discomfort. Our GP prescribed painkillers.

I developed an intermittent pain in my left arm and was hospitalised for one night. The consultant decided it was probably an atypical angina. No heart damage was detected so I was discharged.

Tilly was hospitalised with acute shingles and given morphine for the pain. This paralysed her gut causing severe constipation. She returned home but was sleepless due to the pain. Tilly was hospitalised again and then discharged with strong laxatives. Against medical advice, Tilly decided to have colonic irrigation as the powerful laxatives were not working. After three such treatments the problem was finally cleared.

Tilly emailed Case Co-ordinator Ernie detailing progress made with Roland's independence skills but pointing out those of his limitations that so far appeared intractable:

Hi Ernie,

It is now six months since my active care involvement with Roland started. I thought it might be helpful to give you some feedback of my skills assessment and his development prior to your pending case review.

Roland has made progress in the following areas:

Personal hygiene: like cleaning himself after toileting and taking a shower unsupervised.

Personal care: includes selecting appropriate day and night clothes and dressing himself; identifying dirty clothes and using a washing machine and tumble dryer with some support.

Communication: Roland has learned to use a simple mobile phone to make and receive calls but is still hesitant and monosyllabic in conversation and might not be able to communicate effectively with any helpline or emergency services.

General domestic tasks: include laying the table for meals, washing up including drying and putting away; making his own hot drinks and cereal breakfast; preparing his own packed lunches with some assistance.

Activities: include consulting weekly activity programmes and time schedules; packing his activity bag accordingly together with sorting correct money for activities from cash box.

Diet: Still sticking with his healthy eating programme and displaying dietary awareness and self-discipline; his weight seems to have stabilised at 68 kilos (his starting weight was 124 kilos three years ago which had been his weight for some time previously)

The above requires continuing inbuilt support structures like cue-cards and/or repetitive reinforcement of methods/structures in place. Roland also seeks constant praise and approval for routine tasks performed independently. (e.g., "I have a clean bottom" or "I have made a cup of tea all by myself"). However, some of this may be attention seeking behaviour.

In addition, the above training and practices have highlighted the following weaknesses and vulnerabilities which have so far proved intractable:

Even when doing tasks that he has mastered Roland is very slow in their execution and easily distracted. He loses focus and forgets the steps in the sequencing of activities, as he will sometimes abandon one task half done to start another.

Roland cannot be hurried and is unable to respond appropriately to sudden changes in plans or unexpected events. (even in harmless situations like milk going sour or running out, he loses the confidence to make tea or breakfast). He is even more helpless if equipment malfunctions e.g. if light bulbs blow or computers crash etc. He is very dependent on routines, and items being in familiar places.

Roland can communicate effectively if he feels supported and comfortable, though his topics and utterances may be repetitive and sometimes irrelevant to the ongoing dialogue. However, if upset or in unfamiliar situations he may become tongue-tied and/or incoherent, requiring the patient use of open questions to elicit the issues troubling him. On the other hand, Roland enjoys his day-centre drama activities and has a talent for using exaggerated responses to connect with people and situations. He can swing from tearfulness to hilarity in an instant depending on the responses around him or the effects he wants to create.

Despite an improvement in mobility due to his weight loss, Roland is still prone to injurious falls without warning due to a congenital problem with his right knee joint (displacing patella). Walking is an act of concentration for him, running is dangerous. He uses stairs with extreme deliberation and slowness as he knows the risk of falls. He should not be in public places unaccompanied as he cannot react quickly to such things as oncoming traffic.

He is also vulnerable if mixing with the public alone as he may respond to instructions from strangers if they are sufficiently assertive or appear to be in authority. For the above reasons it is *unsafe for Roland to be out and about unsupported, despite the fact he has a rudimentary awareness of physical risks.*

Although Roland has a concept of personal property, he has little idea of the use and value of money. He would not challenge incorrect change in a shop or on larger scale he has no understanding of general financial management beyond the contents of his piggy bank.

I hope the above report proves useful in assessing Roland's future care needs and placement.   His mother Pat has Alzheimer's Disease and remains detained in hospital under the Mental Health Act. As a result, she will not be able to return to a parenting role, so Robert and I are sharing the caring and sustained efforts to increase Roland's independence skills. Given our ages and recent health issues we would welcome a review and a discussion on supported living options for Roland. I am willing to support the preparation and transition for this next major step but, like Robert, I am unable to continue Roland's care long term. Tilly

In response to an immediate reply from Ernie, Tilly added that she and I considered it necessary to plan for placing Roland in supported living within twelve months – due to our ages and recent/ongoing health issues.

11: Enter the NHS - 2018

The tribunal convened to deal with Pat's request for discharge met in Bellingham House, Bodmin, on 20th April. A QC chaired the proceedings. The professionals were given a detailed report about Pat which I did not see. However, the proceedings were fairly informal, and everyone was invited to speak. It was explained that Pat had declined to attend the tribunal: she was in her nightclothes and pacing up and down the ward in an agitated state. Her solicitor opined that she was not ready for discharge. This was echoed by the lead psychiatrist who added that Pat should continue detained under S.3 of the Mental Health Act for her own safety. The psychiatrist said a costs embargo in Cornwall had been lifted so more nursing homes were now available, but Pat was currently not stable enough for discharge even to the most skilled of homes.

In reply to a question from the Judge, the psychiatrist said Pat's discharge was likely to be months away as Garner Ward needed to be sure that whatever medication regime was arrived at would be effective in stabilizing Pat's behaviour. She said that Pat was becoming more agitated, and when not upset tended to be over-familiar with patients and staff. However, she did not resist taking medication. In any case, continuation of S.117 funding and S.17 leave were recommended. CPN Brenda would be involved in discharge planning. The diagnoses were Alzheimer's Disease with some vascular dementia. I mentioned the progression from mild cognitive impairment after the wrist fracture repair in 2013 through SVD to Alzheimer's in 2015. I also flagged up Pat's worsening eyesight due to cataracts. I praised the care given to Pat in Garner Ward and there was general hilarity when I characterized the atmosphere there as having a Rabelaisian liveliness. The tribunal's decision was that Pat should remain in Garner Ward under S.3 of the MHA at least until it was up for review in June 2018. After the meeting broke up, Pat's solicitor advised me off-the-record that if Pat was placed in a nursing home with S.117 NHS funding and the Clinical Commissioning Group would seek to discontinue funding, it was open to me to request a tribunal hearing and summon a Commissioner to explain the reasons for discontinuance. She said in these circumstances the CCG often caved in and reversed its decision.

In July, Garner Ward rang to say Pat had been found a place at Saltdene House. Tilly and I visited and were shown around. It was adjacent to St Saviours Church, and the place was a large Grade II listed vicarage that had been converted into a care centre. It was labyrinthine inside with many staircases and a variety of spaces – from private rooms for the more able residents to communal lounges and a good-sized dining area. The decorative condition wasn't great, but the place smelt clean, and it was well-staffed by friendly care assistants and nurses.

CPN Brenda rang to say there was to be a review of Pat's placement at Saltdene to decide if the S.17 leave should be discharged. She said this wouldn't affect funding. She added that it was okay for me to attend. At the meeting, discharge of S.17 was agreed. S.117 aftercare funding was to be confirmed, and then reviewed every six months, but likely to be renewed in perpetuity and not means-tested as the only practical alternative to a nursing home for Pat was hospital admission. A nurse said Pat seemed to be settling in well. She was able to drink and feed herself - especially if someone sat with her. She was tactile and compassionate toward other residents. She would do some door-knocking and handle-rattling in the evenings as part of "sundowning behaviour" but this was not excessive. A falls risk was recognized – so Pat was on 2-hourly watch at night.

Tilly and I talked about moving back into the old family home with Roland until Pat passed away – an idea that had popped into my head after visiting Pat while Tilly was seeing relatives in Bristol. Tilly accepted the idea but said it would be essential to maintain the momentum of Roland's independence training and that I might need to take more of a lead with this.

After the evening meal, Tilly and I worked for a few hours in the garden at the old house. I reconnected a hose that ran its length and Tilly did a lot of watering while I tidied generally and shovelled up fallen apples and dead leaves and put them on the compost heaps. I had previously cleared the shed and garage gutters of leaves. It was dark when we finished at 10pm and we stood for a while inside the unlit house. Tilly reaffirmed that she loved the garden and believed that she could be happy living in the house with me and Roland – though she perceived energies there – both in visitation and residual – that would take love and patience to befriend and dispel respectively. As we conversed in this vein, we both felt tingles running up and down our backs. Tilly thought there was a female presence who did not like what had happened to the house, but Tilly hoped that we could make friends and gain her support in making a happy home there.

I received a long phone call from Ian of Cornwall Social Services regarding the Deprivation of Liberty Statement (DOLS) assessment for Pat. He and a doctor had agreed Pat lacked capacity to make her own welfare decisions, but they needed my input. I described the relevant events since September 2015 including my pneumonia and inability to continue caring adequately for her at home. At Ian's request I agreed to be Pat's personal representative (a legal status in the event of Pat wanting to leave Saltdene) which he assured me did not conflict with me also being her "nearest relative" under the Act. He said he would be recommending Pat stay in Saltdene for twelve months before the next review.

12: Options for Roland

At the end of July, Roland had a "well-man" appointment with practice nurse Angela. I raised the question of possible anaemia, but Angela looked up Roland's recent blood test results for haemoglobin, HBA1C, liver, kidney and prostate functions, and found that they were all normal. Angela measured Roland's height, weight and BP. He had lost ten kilograms in the last year and his BP was 117/70. She agreed a sight test would be a good idea as I had noticed Roland's long-distance vision appeared to have deteriorated somewhat. As we were leaving, I saw Dr Maddie who enquired after me and Pat. She knew Pat was in Saltdene House and spontaneously gave me a hug.

I rang Una – leader of the Out and About club about support services. Inter alia she said it was intended that her daughter Debbie would be accommodated with her friend Sally in a house managed by MENCAP. Una advised me to contact MENCAP on Roland's behalf.

Tilly took Roland to the Craft Barn and spoke to manager Wendy about our preference to accommodate Roland at the bungalow with a suitable companion. Wendy agreed with this, also advising against going down the "shared lives" route. I rang MENCAP and obtained contact details regarding their housing scheme.

In a further conversation with Craft Barn staff, I spoke with Amanda and talked about the shared lives project. Although a shared lives provider herself, Amanda agreed that some families lived off the income derived from their LD tenants but treated them little better than lodgers. Amanda added that a Downs guy called Arun, and Roland's younger namesake, were in supported living provision in separate houses. She also mentioned Barry, another Downs guy who had been turfed out of his shared lives accommodation and was presently in residential care. Amanda said she would give Arun's mother Dolly my contact details in case the names of potential sharers with Roland came up. I talked about trying not to leave independent living arrangements for Roland too late - citing my father's death at the age of 72. Amanda replied that she had lost both her grandmother and mother to cancer in their late sixties.

In early September, the weather turned sunny and warm. I mowed the grass at the bungalow while Tilly was delivering Roland to The Craft Barn. On the way, she shopped at Aldi where Roland embarrassed her by play-acting that he would be punished for being naughty by being sent to bed without his supper! When I collected Roland from The Craft Barn I spoke to Wendy and Amanda about a companion for Roland. Amanda had again forgotten to contact Dolly on my behalf but mentioned someone called Steve – a slow-learner in his late 40s (not Downs) who was looking to exit a Shared Lives placement, and someone called Billy - an autistic chap in his thirties who wanted to leave the parental home – though Wendy said his parents were very pleasant people. That evening I took Roland and Tilly drumming – her first session for a while. It was fairly well-attended with some old faces missing but some new ones who had joined which balanced this. We left after the tea break. Tilly said she enjoyed the abbreviated session. Roland

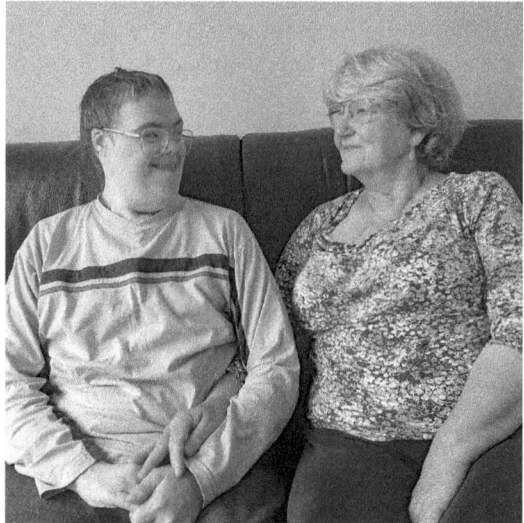

ROLAND AND TILLY: 2019

was keen to be friendly with her to atone for his earlier misbehaviour.

I had a long telephone conversation with Dolly – a retired social worker who had previously been assigned to Roland. Her son Arun was in his 40s and lived in a council house with support for all the hours he spent there – including nights. Dolly also knew other shared lives service users – along with their personal histories and current support arrangements. She gave me the impression that we were receiving less financial help than she would have expected to care for Roland. The upshot of the conversation was that Dolly did not recommend "shared lives" or sharing with a housemate. Struggling to control her feelings, she related some of the difficulties she'd had trying to get and retain adequate support for Arun over the years – despite having inside knowledge of the system. She advised that Tilly and I should push hard for as many agency support hours as possible to help Roland be as independent as he could be at the bungalow.

I spoke to Annie about the plan for Roland to remain at the bungalow. She agreed with Dolly that a housemate might not be the best solution – citing administrative difficulties such as the housemate's financial and support arrangements with the Council and benefits agencies as additional considerations. However, Annie added that the agency she worked for was approved by Cornwall Council as a provider of support services to LD clients at home. I concluded the current plan would have to wait until the old family home was about to become habitable again, then request a bungalow-based home-care review for Roland by Adult Social Care before starting negotiations for a support package.

In mid-October Tilly packed Roland's bags for his Minehead Butlins Holiday with the Craft Barn crew. On his return a week later, we had a debrief from Wendy:

In her and the other Craft Barn carers' assessments, Roland was "nowhere near independent"

He wet himself on an outing and needed to be taken back to his chalet by a carer to change his clothes.

He was inconsistent around personal hygiene – sometimes forgetting to wear his night-pants and on another occasion wandering around with a soiled pair looking for somewhere to dispose of them. On one occasion he left the toilet seat in his shared chalet smeared with faeces but did not attempt to clean it up.

He was un-self-conscious about nudity: stripping off in front of children in the changing area at the swimming pool and leaving the door open while using toilet cubicles. This could cause offence and/or put him at risk of abuse.

He was very slow at food outlets – causing queues to form and potentially irritating other diners. He was resistant to being hurried. When Wendy had chivvied him about the time, he was taking to choose items from the self-service counter he turned to her and said in a very audible voice "I am disabled you know" – to Wendy's considerable embarrassment.

He was mono-syllabic when using his mobile phone – apparently unable to answer questions clearly or describe where he was or what he was doing.

In unfamiliar or stressful situations, he tended to freeze – potentially putting himself at risk if prompt responses were necessary.

He needed a lot of one-to-one support throughout the holiday, or else would stand around looking lost. He was generally slow at getting up, getting dressed and getting ready for activities.

I left a message with the duty social worker for Ernie saying that we needed an assessment for a home care support package. She seemed unaware of Roland's family background and asked a number of questions. I sent an email requesting urgent help from Adult Social Care regarding home care for Roland. Ernie replied saying he would pass the info on.

Social worker Gillian rang to say she'd been allocated to Roland and an appointment was made to see myself and Tilly early in December 2018. She spent an hour and a half with us as we recounted recent family history – with particular reference to Roland and our assessment of his abilities and needs. Although she looked only to be in her twenties, Gillian came across as quite experienced. In response to our proposal that Roland could be supported at the bungalow she doubted that Adult Social Care would sanction the necessary funding. She queried our aversion to the shared lives/fostering scheme then mentioned Hendra Parc as a possible residential option – though she had little information about the place to hand. Tilly and I detailed the progress Roland had made with self-help skills since September 2017 but made it clear that he would need 24/7 supervision to keep him safe. We then emphasized that we could not sustain the current caring regime. Tilly mentioned moving to Manchester to support her son and grandson and I said I would struggle without Tilly to support me. Tilly showed Gillian around the bungalow. As Gillian departed, she said she would call at the Gentian Centre to meet Roland.

Later I rang the Gentian Centre. I spoke to May who said Gillian had spent an hour talking to Roland – who had ranged from monosyllabic to communicative and back again during the session. May added that Roland had become tearful about missing his mum after Gillian had left – but back at the bungalow Roland initially said he would rather go ten-pin bowling with the Gentian Centre than visit Saltdene.

I rang the Gentian centre to say I would be taking Roland to the Saltdene Christmas party, and he would thus miss the bowling that day. Mention of a party had persuaded him.

Discussed with Tilly support options for Roland at the bungalow. Our conclusion was that we could probably manage in the short-term if we had respite Friday to Monday every week – like a weekly Tregarne.

I took Roland to visit Pat at the Saltdene party. They had laid on a buffet and there was a singer who performed Christmas standards. Several children were present – offspring of both staff and visitors – so the atmosphere was more lively than usual. Pat was awake throughout and passed comments – several of which made sense. Speaking to me, she complimented the staff on their cleverness – adding that she found it hard nowadays to work things out and find the right words when speaking. She also said how lovely the toddlers looked. But she didn't seem to recognize Roland as himself. When a nurse gushed about what a nice young man Roland looked, Pat muttered that he didn't look very nice to her! Undeterred, Roland put on a broad grin and stared at his mum. Pat stared back, then slowly drew closer and closer to him – finally kissing his cheek and remarking that he was lovely.

Cornwall Council emailed saying Roland had been granted a renewal of his blue parking badge. I emailed Gillian enquiring about progress with Roland's case, also saying Hendra Parc would not be suitable but scouting the idea of increased respite as an interim measure.

I took Roland for an eye test at Specsavers – his first since 2012. His eyes were pronounced structurally healthy though his right eye remained lazy and short-sighted. Ordered him some spectacles.

2019 began and I continued my weekly visits to see Pat at Saltdene House. I found that evenings were the best as she was more likely to be awake and I had the opportunity to speak to more of the staff if I was there at 8pm when the night shift came on duty. Pat rarely seemed to recognize me but seemed to enjoy the one-to-one attention. In conversation, her choices of words were often bizarre, but I could sometimes guess at her meaning based on facial expression, body language and our long association with each other. The anxiety, agitation and occasional aggression that had been increasingly difficult to manage at home were generally well-controlled by the combination of anti-psychotic drugs she was given. Her wakefulness at night was no problem at Saltdene due to the 24/7 staffing.

I rang social worker Gillian. Whilst acknowledging the budgetary constraints under which Adult Social Care operated, I reiterated my wish that Roland be supported at the bungalow rather than looked after in any other accommodation. Gillian asked if Roland could be left unattended, but I said we were wary of doing this for safety reasons. She suggested it might be worth a try. I then talked about fitting cameras and other security equipment at the bungalow and Gillian replied this might be a possibility. She finished the call by arranging to see Roland at home on 23rd January and at MTL the following day.

Following the conversation with Gillian, I discussed with Tilly the idea of letting Roland spend night hours unattended, providing that security equipment was in place and that someone saw him at bedtime and for breakfast. Tilly was doubtful, saying that if Roland was provided with an alarm system or panic button, she would find it difficult to sleep – expecting it to go off at any moment. I replied that on the contrary it would be a reassuring factor for me.

That evening I visited Pat. She was fairly drowsy throughout but said she was glad to see me. Amid the usual comments on what was happening in the room Pat made a few remarks about love and mortality that were quite poignant. Paraphrasing these, she said it was nice to see people but also sad to say goodbye – knowing that she would have to die sometime soon. Somewhat lamely I suggested she might return – equipped with a new body – but Pat said that she might not meet me again and would miss the cuddles and closeness that we had enjoyed.

On 23rd January Gillian visited and spent some time talking to Roland before involving Tilly and me. We talked around a few options for supporting Roland at the bungalow. Gillian was in favour of equipping Roland with a panic alarm and experimenting with leaving him unattended at the bungalow at different times of day and possibly most of the night. Tilly was doubtful about the latter, but we said we'd reserve judgement until after short absences and the panic alarm had been trialled. Gillian also said she wanted another assessor to gauge Roland's potential for living semi-independently and would arrange this in addition to the referral for an alert system. She also mentioned the option of a care budget that Tilly and I could manage. I commented that whereas Roland could occupy himself with his PlayStation, music etc at the bungalow, his activities and socializing at day centres were also important. I said that in principle I would be willing to subsidize his continued attendance at day centres if his personal budget was reduced due to funding of home care.

A week later, Lifeline installer Ralph successfully installed the telephone equipment, CO and smoke detectors. When Roland returned home, we explained the use of the wrist-worn combined panic button and falls sensor and made a test call. I wasn't sure that Roland grasped the difference between emergency and non-emergency situations though.

Psychologist Dilys rang as a result of a referral from Gillian. She wanted to do baseline tests to establish Roland's level of cognitive functioning as Downs people were more likely to develop dementia with age.

After the evening meal I faffed about with an internet security camera and finally got it sending images to my mobile and the PC at the old house. The panoramic views of Roland's bedroom and the kitchen/diner, both in daylight and at night were excellent, but the two-way

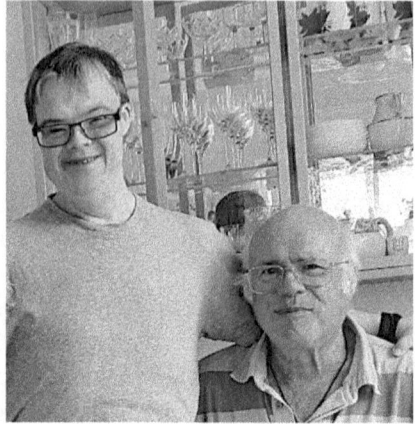

ROLAND AND DAD: 2019

speech facility did not seem to work well due to the delay in refreshing the internet link, though sounds from Roland's room were audible via the PC.

That night, after Roland had settled in bed, I slept at the old family home leaving Roland in the bungalow. I woke at 1.30 am and checked on Roland using the video-link. He was peacefully asleep. Woke again at 6.30 am and he was on his PlayStation. I returned to the bungalow at 7 am and did the usual routines until Roland left for the Gentian Centre.

I tested Roland's response to ringing the doorbell when he knew I was out. He didn't respond although I rang the bell twice a few minutes apart. I praised him for this, then discovered he had left the side door unlocked, presumably when emptying the kitchen bin when the kitchen door was locked. Next, I trialled Roland's response to a power outage affecting his PlayStation. Despite being primed by me to ring me if this happened, he failed to do so - instead staring at his blank TV screen for several minutes before wandering into the kitchen, whereupon I re-entered the bungalow and eventually got him to remember that he should have rung me.

Psychiatrist Dilys arrived at with her trainee and took Tilly and me through a one-hour questionnaire exploring Roland's abilities and limitations. We took the opportunity to say that we had been monitoring Roland sleeping alone at the bungalow since the end of March 2019 but were still concerned that he remained vulnerable to mishaps due to his inability to function appropriately if anything out of the ordinary were to occur. We cited his confusion when we cut power to his play -station and TV, and more importantly, that he wasn't remembering to re-lock the front door when he returned from emptying bins. We were also disappointed at the lack of progress from Adult Social Care in offering home-care options. Dilys said she would keep us in the loop as regards the report she would write after interviewing Roland at MTL and would apprise Gillian of our concern at the lack of progress and the fact that, despite spending my nights at the old house, I was still not sleeping properly due to worrying about Roland's safety and was consequently operating with a continuing sleep-deficit. This latter point was well-emphasized by Tilly.

After Dilys and colleague departed, Tilly and I had a discussion about the way forward in the short term. We concluded that the two of us would probably get more sleep if I was at the bungalow and Tilly was at the old house - as she wasn't getting sufficient sleep either due to being sensitive to my anxieties.

When Tilly and I returned to the bungalow from our excursion to Plymouth we were greeted by Roland informing us that he had gone out into the back garden for a while to enjoy the sunshine. He had locked the external doors on returning indoors but this episode – assuming Roland had indeed gone outside and was not just talking about it – rang an alarm bell with Tilly who felt sure this unusual behaviour (for Roland) was a further indication of inconsistency and thus represented a significant safeguarding issue.

I submitted a claim for Personal Independence Payment (PIP) as Disability Living Allowance was being discontinued.

A false alarm generated by the Lifeline system caused paramedics to enter the bungalow at 4 am using the keysafe. They didn't seem fussed about their wasted journey.

Pat was taken ill at Saltdene, vomiting and shaking then becoming unresponsive. I spent six hours in A&E with her before she was discharged with antibiotics for a suspected chest infection. She perked up on returning to Saltdene.

On the second of August 2019 it was Roland's 43rd birthday. He received a Candy Crush themed tee-shirt and mug from Warren. The day was also marked by bacon sarnies for breakfast, plus a home-baked carrot cake to take to the Gentian Centre. A letter from DWP arrived granting Personal Independence Payment to Roland at an enhanced rate, which was very welcome news. A week later Ernie came to talk about support options for Roland. We re-emphasized the urgency of making suitable arrangements given my and Tilly's age and recent illnesses. We also explained, with examples, why it was unsafe to leave Roland unattended overnight. Ernie said he would come back to us with details and costs of the available options.

Tilly and I discussed our ongoing activities and plans. We agreed that we should continue to push Adult Social Care to provide support for Roland, but that if nothing had materialized by Easter 2020, we would move Roland back to the old family home and give him the first-floor bedroom currently used as Tilly's sewing station. This would entail Roland accepting a smaller room, with all of his currently little-used games and CDs boxed up and stored away, but it would mean we would all have a home together until something more future-oriented could be arranged. At a meeting with Ernie at Morley Tamblyn lodge it was agreed that Roland lacked capacity to make major decisions although he seemed to embrace the idea of moving to supported living. Ernie circulated Roland's details to various residential homes.

At the end of September, following a fall at home and a severe headache, Tilly was referred for neurological tests. An MRI scan showed pinching of the spinal cord in her neck requiring surgery and a long period of recovery.

At the end of October, Virginia – a journalist friend – popped in for a visit. Before she left, she mentioned a friend of hers who had found a MENCAP-managed shared house for her Downs daughter who was younger than Roland. I contacted the friend by email. On her advice I contacted MENCAP, who responded saying a vacancy had arisen in Lostwithiel. I set up lasting powers of attorney (LPAs) both for Health and Welfare and Financial Affairs for me and Warren regarding Roland. By the end of 2019, the bungalow and the old family home had been renovated. We left the bungalow and moved Roland to the family home to await the outcome of his Lostwithiel application, and Tilly sold her property in Landrake.

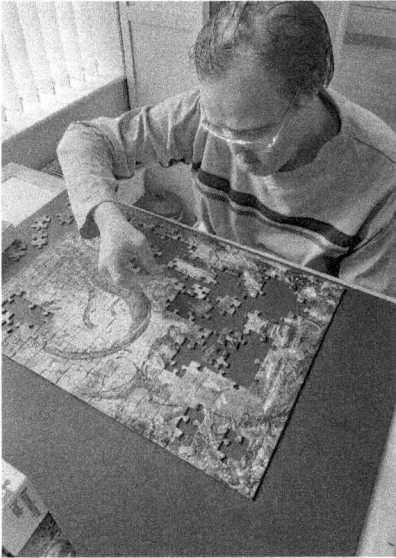

JUNGLE JIGSAW: 2018

13: Mr independent - 2020

Tilly, Roland and I met with Mencap managers at the bungalow. There was a subsequent meeting between the managers, Tilly and me at the Lostwithiel centre which was an old-style seven bedroom detached house standing in its own grounds. Roland was then invited to visit. We all liked the place and its staff and residents.

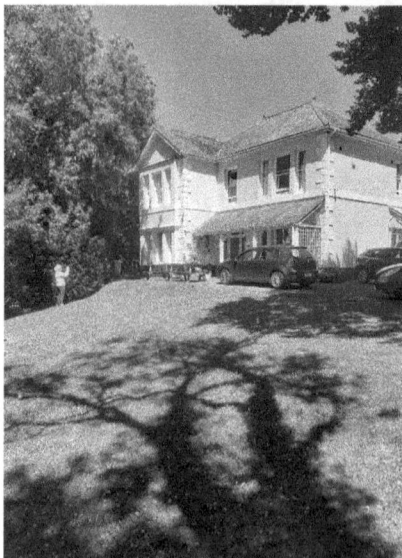

THE LOSTWITHIEL CENTRE

March brought the beginning of the coronavirus pandemic, and all day centres were closed.

Tilly underwent surgery in April as the pandemic was worsening. The operation was successful, and she was discharged the next day to minimize the risk of COVID19 infection, which in her vulnerable condition would have been fatal.

I wrote to a senior manager in Adult Social Care asking them to fund the placement for Roland, pointing out that Tilly and I could no longer cope with his care due to health issues. To our joy and relief, funding for Roland's Lostwithiel placement was granted shortly afterwards.

On 30th of July 2020 Roland tested negative for coronavirus and was allowed to move into his new home at Lostwithiel. For his 44th birthday on the 2nd of August 2020, his new housemates organized a barbecue which we all enjoyed.

Although Housing Benefit was to be applied for by MENCAP, I was informed by the DWP that I was the responsible person regarding Roland's ESA, PIP and UC and thus needed appointee status with the DWP so that they would be authorized to talk to me about Roland's benefits. I therefore went through the necessary processes to obtain appointeeships.

In October, back in Saltash, Tilly's laptop made a notification sound even though it was switched off. This was the latest in a series of electrical anomalies over the previous few weeks, including the cordless phones chirping in their cradles without being touched, and the cooker cooling fan either failing to switch off or switching on from cold. Tilly was apprehensive that all these phenomena presaged a traumatic event, but she was unable to clarify the sensing. Events were to prove her right.

We continued to visit Roland at Lostwithiel regularly until barred by the national lockdown early in November.

14: Emergency and Recovery

On 22nd November we had a call to say Roland had been found at breakfast time sitting on the floor next to his bed with a bump on his head near his left eye. His speech and movement were impaired, so an ambulance took him to the Royal Cornwall Hospital at Treliske, Truro. Staff member Charmaine followed him to A&E.

I Spoke to A&E Dr Trevecca. He broke the shocking news that a CT scan had revealed a bleed on the right-hand side of Roland's brain i.e., a haemorrhagic stroke. His left arm and leg were motionless, and he was not speaking. Early in the evening Roland was admitted to Phoenix Ward where he was seen by stroke specialist Dr Brady. She made it clear that Roland's condition was potentially life-threatening, and that if there was evidence of brain swelling due to further bleeding the options were to have an emergency hemi-craniectomy to relieve the pressure or let Roland die. Further, such surgery could not reverse the damage already caused by the bleed. In reply to her question, I said that, if I were in Roland's shoes, I wouldn't want my life to be prolonged if that meant I would remain severely mentally and physically impaired with no prospect of recovery.

Late in the evening Tilly drove me to Treliske, finally reaching the hospital at midnight. There we were told only one bedside visitor was allowed, for a maximum of one hour. I had to don an apron and surgical gloves as well as my mask to enter Phoenix ward where I also had to sign a form and have my temperature taken. Roland was awake but drowsy, answering simple questions by nodding, shaking his head or giving a thumbs-up with his right hand. His left arm and leg had no movement. It was very difficult for him to vocalize but he did manage to whisper, "I want the toilet". I reassured him this wasn't a problem as he was wearing absorbent pants. Dr Brady had also mentioned impaired kidney function which was unexplained. Roland was on a 125ml/hour fluid drip as he was unable to swallow. He was also receiving coagulant and anti-convulsive medication intravenously. He seemed uncomfortable lying on his left side, so I asked the nurse to turn him onto his back, whereupon he went to sleep shortly before 1 a.m.... my leaving time.

The following day I rang Phoenix Ward and was told a doctor's report was expected after lunch. Roland had apparently spent a fairly comfortable night. I rang Warren and talked around all Roland's health issues. Rang Phoenix ward again at 4pm. Staff nurse Olga consulted doctor's notes and said that there was currently no evidence of further bleeding or of raised blood pressure. Roland had become a little more responsive and physios had made an initial assessment. The impaired kidney function was being investigated. Blood tests were being done and a kidney ultrasound had been booked. Olga explained that the one-hour visits were only being permitted because Roland was in a high dependency unit, and visitors had to be from the same household bubble. I phoned Warren and relayed all this info.

George, the locum manager at Lostwithiel, rang offering support. I felt rather low but better than when news of Roland's stroke had first broken.

Off to Treliske after breakfast. I waited at reception while Tilly visited Roland. She reported back that he beamed on recognizing her and managed to say her pet name "Twinkletoes". His tongue and left knee were severely swollen. The left-hand side of his face, and his left arm and leg remained paralysed, though when Tilly placed her hand on the right-hand side of his head, his left arm and leg had twitched twice. The hydration and glucose drip were discontinued in favour of a tube into his stomach. Nurses asked for Roland's dressing gown and pyjamas so he could spend time in a chair.

Back home, George rang and asked for a progress report. Alan from Treliske's LD team made contact. Checked with Phoenix ward who confirmed only Tilly and I could visit. I informed Warren.

On 25th November we set off for Treliske via Lostwithiel, where we collected Roland's pyjamas and dressing gown. At Treliske, while Tilly waited in the car, I met with Dr Brady, nurses Nancy and Vanessa (who mentioned she had a brother with Downs Syndrome), Sybil from the LD support team, physio Jasmine and a team of urologists. Roland's inability to urinate normally was causing concern as it was harming his kidneys. So, after a failed attempt to catheterize him in the normal way, a supra-pubic catheter was inserted directly into his bladder via his abdominal wall under a local anaesthetic. Roland bore the discomfort of this procedure well and half a litre of urine was quickly drained. Afterwards Roland gave a thumbs up to the surgeons and patted one of them on the back. I was issued with a "carer's passport" to facilitate future visits. I was with Roland for nearly four hours and when I left, he gave a valedictory wave with his good hand.

Back home I gave Warren, George and the Lostwithiel team an update. Also rang Ernie who had been unaware of Roland's illness.

Two days later we returned to Treliske. Tilly spent an hour and a half with Roland who seemed a little more alert and able to take some yoghurt by mouth. Tilly face-timed Warren so he could see Roland who apparently recognized him. They were pleased to see each other. We left a request on the Matthew Manning spiritual healing website (to which we had been subscribers prior to Roland's illness) for Roland to receive absent healing.

Warren rang. We talked about Roland's illness, general family matters and mortality, including the advisability of keeping one's affairs in order and leaving notes and instructions for loved ones.

I woke around 5.30 am on 29th with my left thumb twitching – reminiscent of a morse code rhythm. This went on for about 30 minutes then stopped as abruptly as it had started. I wondered if it had something to do with the requested absent healing.

In the meantime, Roland had been moved to a less high-dependency area of Phoenix ward. He seemed comfortable, drifting in and out of a doze but rousing whenever there was activity nearby and responding with nods and shakes of head to questions. A male doctor took me aside and showed me the CT scan image of Roland's brain. A white blob was clearly visible, indicating the area damaged by the bleed. The doctor said that its cause was possibly a spike in blood pressure, but that Roland's BP had reverted to normal. In reply to my question the doctor said the dead nerve cells would not regenerate but that the brain might compensate to some extent by finding different motor nerve pathways, but that this process could take several weeks. Back at Roland's bedside, a nurse was spooning in yoghurt. She told me Roland was a very good patient and that they had taken him to the hospital shop in a wheelchair and bought him a Rudolf Reindeer soft toy. I thanked them. Two physios arrived and examined Roland's knees. The swelling had gone down, and his tongue also looked normal. One of the physios asked Roland to lift his left knee. To my pleased surprise he did so. The doctor returned and checked Roland's chest, heart and urine tube – all okay. He said there was a plan to transfer Roland to the stroke rehabilitation unit at Bodmin Hospital.

That evening we joined in Matthew Manning's online mass healing event at 7pm. I focused my thoughts on Roland, though I also thought of Pat. Tilly chose to sit downstairs for the same hour, also concentrating on sending healing energies to Roland.

The next day we returned to Treliske. Tilly spent nearly two hours in the ward. However, things were not quite so positive as on the previous day. Tilly met with Dr Brady and the physios. Roland had been allocated a bed at the Bodmin stroke rehab unit and was due to be transferred there at 3pm. However, tests still showed an elevated white cell count which, together with a rise in blood pressure, prompted the medics to delay Roland's move until the results of further tests were in. Roland added to their caution by confiding to Tilly that his chest hurt. He presented as rather drowsy and took a while to register her arrival. Encouraged by his ability to sit up in bed unaided despite his left arm showing no sign of movement, the physios tried him standing but his left leg could not bear his weight. This upset Roland, but Tilly comforted him.

On 1st December I made a solo visit to Treliske and saw the speech therapist and consultant Dr Brady. Roland was fairly drowsy throughout, but the speech therapist got him to say a few words and attempt a rendering of "silent night" plus encouraging him to feed himself most of a small pot of yoghurt. Dr Brady said Roland's ability to move his left leg was improving though there was no movement yet in his left arm. His heart was all right, his kidneys were recovering, and his lung function was okay. X-rays showed no infection in his lungs, but he needed a CT scan to check if there were any small blood clots. If there were no clots found he could move out of the "acute" ward.

The next day I drove Tilly to Treliske. She spent just over an hour with Roland and spoke to a doctor, speech therapist and physio. Roland seemed a little brighter, speaking more and feeding himself some yoghurt. When trying to move his left arm on request his left leg moved instead. The physio took this to be a positive indication and initiated some passive exercises for the left arm to stimulate sensory nerves. The latest CT scan showed no clots in his lungs, so he was passed fit for transfer to the Woodfield stroke rehab unit at Bodmin later in the day.

Back home, George rang, and I gave him the latest news. At 7pm there was a call from Bodmin to say Roland had arrived and was watching television.

In the afternoon of the fourth, we collected some clothes from Lostwithiel then took them to Bodmin Hospital. We were met outside by physio June who was part of Roland's care team in the stroke rehab unit. She was very pleasant but reiterated the hospital's policy of excluding all visitors during the pandemic. Roland was in a private room on the ground floor of the facility. We looked in through the window and he gave us a lop-sided grin and a wave. He seemed alert and cheerful. They had got him to stand with support and were pleased with his progress in the short time since he'd arrived the previous evening.

On 7th December Dulcie rang from Lostwithiel and introduced herself as the new manager. She asked after Roland. I said he was in the stroke rehab unit at Bodmin and that they thought there would be permanent damage as a result of the stroke, but that physios Nobby and June would be working to restore what function they could. They were currently concentrating on Roland's left leg which had lost muscle tone to the extent that the knee-cap was slipping out of position, which was the same issue Roland permanently had with his right knee. I asked about Roland's future at the shared house and Dulcie said it would depend on his level of recovery and additional support from Adult Social Care.

We visited at Bodmin, and Roland was wheeled out into a sunny patio area wrapped in blankets and with his anti-thrombosis stockings and nose tube still in place. Although he looked tired, he was alert. In the course of making conversation, I reminded him his mum had been in Garner Ward at Bodmin. Typical of Roland, he mis-heard Garner as banana and was highly amused when I corrected him. He said that he'd had yoghurt at breakfast and managed to spoon in some mushy peas at lunchtime. We didn't stay more than twenty minutes because it was cold despite the sunshine. Roland looked pleased when I handed his Asus tablet to a nurse – who said there was wi-fi in the rooms.

Two days later I rang Bodmin Hospital and spoke to Dr Susan. She said that there were no immediate general health concerns with Roland but that she would note his file with the need to review his urination issues.

On our next visit we handed over Roland's favourite red blanket and met with physio Nobby outside. He said his team were making progress with restoring function to Roland's left leg and were prioritising this over his left arm, as leg strength was important for being able to get up from a seated position and maintain a standing position. Nobby returned to Roland's room and demonstrated how Roland could voluntarily move his left hip, knee and ankle joints to order. His left arm was still floppy, but Nobby said they had seen flickers of movement in the shoulder and elbow joint. As far as I could tell from talking to him through the partially opened window, Roland seemed alert and in reasonable spirits. Nobby commented that Roland was popular on the ward due to his friendly and positive attitude and that he seemed to be doing his best to engage with the physio exercises even though these were tiring for him.

Speech therapist Jade said Roland was now being given more solid food which he was managing well. The nose tube had been retained to administer medication and because swallowing fluids still made him cough. Jade added that Roland's speech and communication was improving. I then spoke to physio June who said that, with the aid of a support frame, Roland had managed a five-metre and two ten-metre walks. The physios' next target was to improve Roland's mobility to the level that he would be able to get from bed or chair to a standing position without needing a hoist. Roland's left knee still required strapping and his left arm was still floppy, but the special walking frame compensated for the latter weakness.

The next day we drove to Bodmin Hospital and briefly greeted Roland through his window, handing over the requested shower gel and toothbrush batteries, then curtains were drawn as he used the toilet. When he had been "re-assembled" we were invited to observe him walking twenty metres along a corridor and back, flanked by physio June and two nurses. He was in good spirits, and it was clear his left leg was bearing his weight and helping to push him along. His left arm showed very little movement but appeared to be contributing somewhat to the stability of his stance. Tilly and I praised him for his impressive efforts – as did the medical staff.

After lunch on 17th, we drove to Bodmin hospital for a window visit. Roland had been moved to a larger ward with other patients and was sitting in a chair, still with his nose tube and anti-thrombosis leggings in place. However, a nurse said he was almost eating normally and had a valve fitted to his urinary catheter instead of a dangling bag, so he could ask for urine to be drained off when his bladder filled. There was also progress with walking. Although we didn't witness it, we were told he could walk with the aid of a tripod stick rather than a walking frame. Roland was very pleased to see us, and to receive a supply of bananas. Tilly clapped her hands to applaud Roland's efforts and he mimicked this, his left arm now able to move at will, though his left hand looked limp. We came away feeling encouraged by how much left-side function he had regained.

Physio June rang around 4pm. She said Roland was continuing to make progress with his mobility and had managed to walk ten metres using only an ordinary walking stick for support, while an assistant was present in case of a stumble. His left kneecap had re-located itself and no longer needed strapping.

Movement and control of his left arm and hand had also improved. He had also enjoyed making some dance moves to music. Roland was regaining his appetite and was disappointed to be given porridge when he could see someone else enjoying a full English breakfast. So, he would be offered skinless sausages for breakfast henceforth! June took a note to liaise with the urology team at Treliske regarding a treatment plan. She said arrangements would be made to meet with staff at Lostwithiel to organize things for Roland's return.

In response to government announcements of further restrictions due to a second wave of Coronavirus infections, I discussed with Warren and family the impact of these changes on proposed in-house get-togethers on 23rd and 27th December. We tentatively considered meeting outdoors somewhere instead so as to include a visit to Roland.

On 20th December we made a window visit to Roland en-famille. With a little help from a nurse, he opened his Get Well Soon card and was also pleased to receive a couple of bananas, although we could see a supply near his bed. Roland still had his nose tube, but Tilly said his anti-thrombosis stockings had gone. Although there seemed to be little strength in his left hand he could articulate his shoulder, elbow and wrist joint and wriggle the fingers of his left hand. He seemed as pleased with this latest progress as we were. In reply to our questions, he said he'd had porridge for breakfast then roast chicken and vegetables for lunch. We left when a nurse started to set up a video for Roland and the two other patients in his room.

Occupational therapist Tania rang. She said the facilities at Lostwithiel, including the stairlift, looked sufficient for Roland – though he would need more one-to-one care hours. She added that his swivel chair should be supplemented by a normal chair with arms to help him when standing up. Roland had also asked for his Christmas jumper and a hat.

Shortly after breakfast on 23rd we set out for Bodmin, arriving shortly before Warren and family. Favoured by a break in the rain, we all gathered around Roland's window and handed over his cards and jumper. After twenty minutes or so we took our leave. Roland had been very happy to see us.

Next to Seaton beach where we had hot drinks at the café before walking along the beach and sea wall. The river had carved eight-foot sand cliffs which Warren enjoyed jumping down and clawing his way back up. The rain returned so we turned back as Charlie and Mitzi were getting wet and cold. At the café we had hot snacks before going our separate ways. It had been great to meet with Warren and family who all seemed well.

Tamara from Bodmin Hospital rang inviting us to an online discharge planning meeting on 30th December, to be attended by members of the hospital rehab team, a Lostwithiel rep and case co-ordinator Ernie.

On Christmas morning we set off for Bodmin. The roads were very quiet, and we arrived to find the ward curtains drawn. After ringing the ward, I handed over Roland's Christmas stocking then waited until 11am when whatever goings-on in Roland's ward concluded and the curtains were pulled back. Roland was seated in a chair near the window having his Christmas jumper put on. He was pleased to see us and enjoyed taking the items in his stocking out one by one. It was immediately noticeable that his nose tube had gone – though he still needed the anti-thrombotic leggings. A nurse said he was eating fairly normally and had done some walking without support, plus his left arm and hand continued to improve. I congratulated the staff on Roland's progress and the nurse said a lot of it depended on Roland concentrating on getting better, which he was doing.

On 28th we visited Roland at Bodmin around 11am. The high spot was when he got up from his chair unaided and walked over to the window! We congratulated him and handed over some bananas and grapes. We didn't stay long as a cold northerly breeze was blowing into the ward from the open window.

On 30th December, the pre-discharge conference call was held with Bodmin hospital staff, plus Dulcie and Ziggy from Mencap. Ernie from Adult Social Care was invited but didn't attend. Roland answered questions when asked. His discharge date was dependent on continued progress and admin issues between Adult Social Care and Mencap being sorted. Decisions were:

Emergency and Recovery

The NHS would not discharge Roland from hospital care until he was fit enough and would continue to provide support after discharge: dietetics, after-stroke monitoring, speech and language therapy, mobility and dexterity therapies, occupational therapy and changing catheter dressing etc – via a community support team.

Medication: paracetamol, omeprazole and others involved with reducing stroke risk.

A urology treatment plan was required. In the meantime, Roland would be instructed how to drain his urine bag and use a commode in his room.

Roland was now walking without support, but he needed supervision, especially when using stairs. There were actions on me to deliver his wheelchair to Bodmin and a dining chair to Lostwithiel – the latter to supplement his swivel chair.

Roland was now eating and drinking nearly normally. Progress was expected to continue, particularly with the use of his left hand.

Anti-thrombotic leggings still required until further notice.

At the end of the meeting, I took the opportunity to thank all the staff for their excellent work with Roland. Dulcie asked my permission for Roland to be vaccinated against COVID – I agreed.

After lunch on 2nd January, I extricated Roland's wheelchair from the garage, cleaned it up and took it to Bodmin hospital where we also did a window visit. Roland was resting on his bed when we arrived, but he got up unaided and walked to a chair near the window. He again seemed very pleased to see us.

Two days later prime minister Boris Johnson announced another, stricter lockdown. No window visits were allowed at Bodmin until further notice. This was disappointing. I asked the nurse to explain our absence to Roland.

On the 7th January I rang Bodmin Hospital. A nurse said Roland was continuing generally to progress very well, especially with eating and walking with minimal supervision. He had dispensed with the anti-thrombotic leggings. A visit to Lostwithiel was planned for the following week. His urine catheter was to remain in place until further notice.

On the 15th, physio Nobby rang from Bodmin Hospital to say Roland was on course to return to Lostwithiel in four days' time following a successful visit. He added Roland had been a model patient and made one of the most complete recoveries from a stroke he had seen. Issues remained re urology and maintaining personal hygiene when toileting, but Roland would have regular visits from an NHS team to help with these. Dulcie emailed to say she was pleased to meet Roland on his home visit and that he looked very well.

Dulcie rang to say Adult Social Care had agreed funding of a six-week transitional support package and that Roland would be returning to Lostwithiel the following day. She recommended we delay our window visit until the 24th. She also agreed it would be OK to deliver Roland's Christmas presents, cash for food and some pineapple jam late that morning.

15: Home Again 2021

So, we went to Lostwithiel after a pleasant sunlit drive taking the usual forty minutes. After handing over the agreed items, we peered through the lounge window. Roland was sitting in an armchair. He turned, smiled and waved. He looked healthy and contented.

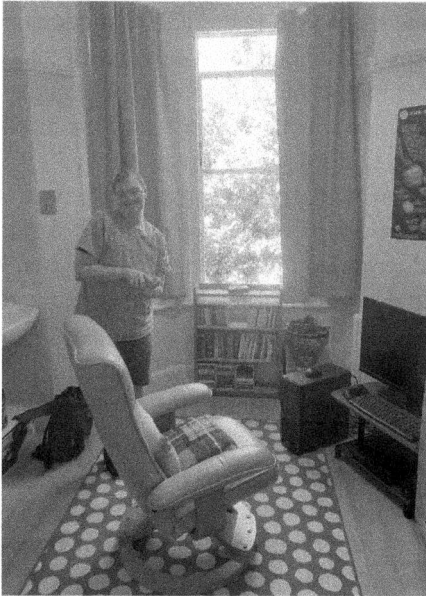

ROLAND'S ROOM AT
THE LOSTWITHIEL CENTRE: 2020

On the 27th January, Dulcie rang again. She said Roland was doing well and was being assisted by visiting NHS staff together with house staff. She said his urology was under review and treatment at Treliske was under discussion. Dulcie added that his Treatment Escalation Plan (TEP) form was also due for a review. His situation regarding state benefits was being looked at by MENCAP administrator Aluna. I explained that his ESA was still being paid to me, out of which I was paying towards the costs of Roland's food etc. I thought that Roland might be migrated to Universal Credit when ESA was phased out but had seen no correspondence about this. PIP had stopped when Roland went to live at Lostwithiel. Dulcie copied me and Ziggy into an email to Roland's new GP regarding a TEP form review.

At the end of January, Aluna emailed asking which benefits Roland received and offering to help with an application for Housing Benefit. I accepted, reflecting that it was just as well I had kept records of my dealings with benefits agencies dating back to Roland's childhood.

Early in February Dulcie emailed saying staff and residents had given Roland a belated Christmas party which he had enjoyed. The following day she rang to discuss getting Roland some straight-leg trousers and hand towels to facilitate management of his urine bag and drying after washes, because Roland's left hand remained weaker than his right. Tilly asked if staff could check Roland's wardrobe for suitable trousers as she was confident there were some pairs already there. She added that we were happy to deliver a supply of hand towels plus additional trousers, along with wet wipes and so on if needed. Dulcie added that she enjoyed her interactions with Roland and said all residents had now received the Oxford AstraZeneca vaccine.

After a further conversation with staff member, Aubrey, we delivered extra trousers, towels, soap and deodorant for Roland. He was pleased to see us and wriggled the fingers of his left hand to show he was regaining full use of it. Aubrey confirmed Roland was able to enjoy his PlayStation again and was doing exercises with play-dough aimed at improving the opposability of his left thumb. Aubrey added that he would be organizing Zoom drama sessions with drama teacher Sue.

A couple of days later, Dulcie rang to say a revised TEP form had been completed for Roland – requiring paramedics to make their best efforts to resuscitate him in the event of a collapse.

In mid-February I rang Roland and Tilly and I spoke with him for about ten minutes. He sounded pleased to hear from us and quite cheerful.

I had telephone conversations with agents Donna and Mary from the DWP regarding Roland's claim for Universal Credit which was to supplement his ESA. They explained that Roland was in the "support group" and would not have to commit to seeking work. Mary confirmed PIP had been suspended as Roland was not self-funding, though it appeared that this decision was under review as part of a rationalisation of Roland's benefits package. I obtained login details for his new web-based UC account and took an action to check the "to-do" tab regularly.

Afterword

I started writing this afterword in September 2021, with local coronavirus infections at a lower level following an ongoing national vaccination campaign. We were looking forward to a long-awaited relaxation of visiting restrictions and social distancing rules.

To all appearances, following his discharge from hospital, Roland slotted back into his Lostwithiel home life as if he'd never been away. He continues to get on very well with his fellow residents and is popular with staff and support workers. Indoor visits are not encouraged so Tilly and I time our trips to coincide with good weather when we can sit outside with Roland in the pleasant garden at Lostwithiel or take him out for meals and occasional shopping trips.

During a visit shortly after his return, Roland was playing boule on the lawn with one of his housemates, umpired by a staff member. He seemed pleased we were visiting and sat at the picnic table with us for a little while, but soon resumed his game – turning to look at us for applause whenever he won. Tilly and I reflected afterwards that, although it felt a little odd to switch roles from parent and full-time carer to visitor, this was exactly the shift that needed to happen if Roland's security is to be assured for the long term.

In summer 2021 we took Roland to Saltash for lunch, then to a Dartmoor Farm for an evening concert staged by Roland's favourite folk band – Seventh Wave Music. He enjoyed the outing but was pleased at being welcomed back to his Lostwithiel home shortly after midnight.

Fast forward to 2022 and day services have resumed. Manager Dulcie left to pursue her career elsewhere but she laid the groundwork for Roland to accompany some of his fellow residents to a day centre further west in Cornwall, and he is now enjoying this new placement. Some of his housemates were already regaining access to outside activities and it was important for Roland's mental and emotional well-being that he didn't miss out on social interaction outside the Lostwithiel Centre, especially as he had become quite close to several of his fellow service users at day centres over many years. It took a while to sort transport arrangements and funding but eventually these issues were ironed out.

Nationally, expenditure on the NHS and particularly geriatric and special needs care is a thorny issue. The country has had to borrow vast sums to sustain the impact of the pandemic and the government will have to grapple with servicing the debt. Increased taxation of both personal income and capital appears inevitable and it remains to be seen whether state and local benefits and allowances will be frozen, reduced, or qualification made more difficult.

Downs Syndrome, and the rights of unborn children with this and other disabling conditions, has been in the news. In July 2021, a High Court action was started to challenge the law that allows Downs' pregnancies to be terminated up to full term – as opposed to the normal twenty-four week time limit for abortions. The action did not succeed but the debate continues.

In a positive development, the Down Syndrome Bill received royal assent in April 2022. It aims to enhance the legal rights of people with Downs Syndrome across several areas of their lives.

This brings the story of my son, Roland, and our wider family to an end for the time being. Thankfully, apart from Pat, we are all in as good health as age and stage allow us to be. Roland is being treated to reduce the risk of post-stroke epileptic episodes but is otherwise doing well, and he is happy in his home. Tilly and I hope the Story of Roland will be useful to those of you who find yourself having to care for a child with Downs Syndrome. In some ways, the biggest problem is dealing with the authorities, both in respect of getting the financial benefits to which Downs people and their families are entitled, and in finding suitable accommodation when needed. This is especially important these days, in view of the fact that these children now live a goodly lifespan and are likely to outlive their parents.

Tilly and I thank our lucky stars – and Roland's – for all the support received to date - both human and financial. However, for all parents and carers of children and adults with Downs Syndrome, the continued importance of engaging with government agencies and Adult Social Care, and of being persistent in ascertaining entitlements and pushing for support, cannot be overstated.

Index

www.ingramcontent.com/pod-product-compliance
Lightning Source LLC
Chambersburg PA
CBHW052138270326
41930CB00012B/2931